PROBLEMATISING YOUNG PEOPLE

PROBLEMATISING YOUNG PEOPLE

A Critical Ethnographic Investigation of ADHD

BY

CHARLES MARLEY
University of Edinburgh, UK

emerald PUBLISHING

United Kingdom – North America – Japan – India – Malaysia – China

Emerald Publishing Limited
Howard House, Wagon Lane, Bingley BD16 1WA, UK

First edition 2020

Reprints and permissions service
Contact: permissions@emeraldinsight.com

British Library Cataloguing in Publication Data
A catalogue record for this book is available from the British Library

ISBN: 978-1-83867-896-8 (Print)
ISBN: 978-1-83867-895-1 (Online)
ISBN: 978-1-83867-897-5 (EPub)

Printed and bound by CPI Group (UK) Ltd, Croydon, CR0 4YY

ISOQAR REGISTERED

ISOQAR certified Management System, awarded to Emerald for adherence to Environmental standard ISO 14001:2004.

Certificate Number 1985
ISO 14001

INVESTOR IN PEOPLE

For Anna, Aonghus and Georgia

Contents

List of Figures

About the Author

Charles Marley has been part of the Section of Clinical Psychology at the University of Edinburgh since 2010. He is currently the Programme Director for the MSc in Mental Health of Children and Young People: Psychological Approaches. His research is interested in the application of critical theory to children and young people's mental health and well-being and focuses on how cultural, political and economic factors interact with local contextual factors to inform the everyday practices regarding children and young people's mental health and well-being.

Preface

Overview of the Investigation

The investigation presented in this book utilised an ethnographic approach, and the scholarship of Michel Foucault, João Biehl, Nikolas Rose and Carol Bacchi to reconnect the wider social, political and institutional factors that were influential in the formation of a particular form of ADHD-related health care. By utilising various strands of their theoretical and empirical material, the investigation aimed to reconnect the nexus of elements that conditioned the possibility for the everyday social practice of ADHD to be in place within an NHS region in Scotland in the present moment.

An overarching aim was to consider ADHD from outside its dominant biomedical explanation by examining the wider context and processes that conditioned the possibility for the emergence of a local social practice of ADHD diagnosis and treatment. The investigation made use of the ethnographic approach of *Vita: Life in a Zone of Social Abandonment* as a methodological guide. *Vita* reconnects the nexus of elements – the 'invisible machinery' – that allowed for the subject of the project to be represented as mentally defective in the present. This project attempts a similar methodological reconnection of the invisible machinery that conditioned the present, but with the social practice of ADHD as the focus.

The analytic approach made use of the concept of 'problematisation', which captures a two-stage process – the questioning of how and why certain 'things' become a problem, but also how these 'things' are shaped as the objects that they become. Objects are not considered as things that previously did not exist being created by discourse, but as things that become what they are because of their interconnected 'apparatus' – the totality of discursive and non-discursive elements that introduce them into the play of true and false. The object of interest for this project was 'young people' and how they were problematised and shaped as the target of certain knowledges. It was through this process, the *how* of their construction as a problem, that the project made the connections that provided the authority for particular problem explanations to be installed as 'real' over other possibilities.

The fieldwork was conducted in a small geographical region in Scotland and consisted of several periods in health and education services. Along with extended periods in these domains, further ethnographic tools utilised included observation of clinical appointments, document analysis, interviews and archival research. Multiple sources of information formed the qualitative data for the investigation, including audio recordings/transcription of clinical appointments, clinical case notes, health service management team meetings and health and education policies and guidelines. The different layers of qualitative material – from individual appointment to national policy – allowed for reconnection of the discursive field in which the current practice of ADHD emerged. The material was engaged with horizontally and vertically within and across the different layers of material, allowing for the examination of the changing discursive background and the problematisation of young people within education and health domains. The analysis revealed discontinuity in how the 'problem' of young people was constructed across time, what was legitimated as solution to these problems, what effects were created and what followed from these effects.

The study is considered a Foucauldian-inspired ethnographic 'case study'. The thesis uses the various chapters to construct a genealogical account of the emergence of the local social practice of ADHD, one that maps and makes visible the multiplicity of events implicated in the construction of young people as particular types of problems and which conditioned the possibility for the social practice of ADHD to become the current means by which young people become known as problems. The account offered provides a theoretical redescription of the rise of ADHD diagnosis and treatment locally, one that aims to trouble accepted explanations by revealing the wider complex network from which the social practice emerged.

Connecting Analysis across Chapters

In Chapters 1 and 2, I establish the frame of reference for this investigation and outline the methodological plan that guided the investigation in the field. Chapter 1 is offered in place of a 'literature review'. My rationale for not providing a 'review' of the ADHD literature is because I take the position that reviewing this material would be nothing more than a reproduction of the 'scientific truth value' of ADHD. Rather than viewing the material as providing access to a 'real' account of ADHD, I consider it as constructing a rhetorical truth value, based on an enactment of procedures of objectivity, that provides ADHD its authority and which allows it to remain a dominant way of constructing young people considered problematic. Instead, what is offered in place of a literature review is a brief account of the positivist literature and an expansion of the ontological and epistemological grounds for the rejection of this literature. The remainder of the chapter provides an account of the theory and concepts that underpin the approach that guided this investigation. This theoretical account is then expanded in Chapter 2, which is presented in two sections. In the first section, I expand the theoretical account, providing a detailed theorising of the main analytical concept that guides the investigation – the apparatus. The concept is then placed within an account of methodological precautions and analytical steps. In the second section of Chapter 2, I provide a detailed account of the procedures for enactment of the theoretical account offered in first part of the chapter.

In Chapter 3, I provide an overview of the changing politico-economic background of the region and the changing requirements of the young person within the new societal order that emerged from this process. The chapter documents the decline of industry in the region; the removal of traditional forms of employment for young people in the area; and the emergence of technologies for disciplining young people towards active citizenship, a form of subjectivity in which the young person would self-improve through vocationally focused learning in order to 'fit' with the emerging post-industrial society. This chapter was made possible by the analytical focus that informed Chapter 4: specifically, the emergence of disadvantage and poverty as a strategic aim the apparatus of education, something that was prominent throughout my discussions with educational professionals in the region. Its visibility in discussions took the form of accounts of the impact of disadvantage locally and 'on' the behaviour of children. These discussions connected to my consideration of 'additional support needs' and its role in solving the impact the 'problem' of 'social exclusion' and 'disadvantage' had on learning. My previous unquestioning acceptance of local disadvantage was disrupted through a conversation with an educational professional, which was made possible by the critical focus on social exclusion in Chapter 4. As such, there was a requirement to extend the critical focus further to understand some of the elements that conditioned the possibility of the problems social exclusion came to represent. The chapter is presented in two sections: one section is offered as a genealogical/topological account of the elements considered important in conditioning outcomes and effects implicated in the emergence of the local procedures of ADHD and a second section where the effects are considered in detail.

The analysis in Chapter 4 was situated within educational sites and documents the conditions that allowed for psychiatric knowledge to play a role within the school. The chapter considers the changing discursive background of 'learning disability', the emergence of the category of Additional Support Needs from within this discursive space, the role this category played in constructing young people as requiring 'support to learn' and how this opened up a discursive space in which psychiatric knowledge and technologies would function. This chapter was made possible by the analysis in Chapter 5: one of the pressing issues, and one that offered legitimacy to the procedures that allowed for psychiatric knowledge to become dominant in CAMHS, was the 'problem' of increased referrals from schools. The question in this chapter was to understand what was 'done' with regard to problems in school and to understand what conditioned the possibility for ADHD to become a solution. As with the previous chapter, this chapter is presented in a similar way: a genealogical/topological account of the elements considered important in conditioning outcomes and effects and a more detailed consideration of these effects.

The analysis in Chapter 5 documents the shifting explanation for young people's behaviour within the Child and Adolescent Mental Health Service (CAMHS) through analysis of clinical case files and team meeting minutes. The analysis documents the conditions that allowed for the emergence of the everyday practice of ADHD within CAMHS, connects this to wider shifting health and education reforms and highlights how this was able to connect to the local schools through the concept/policy agenda of 'well-being promotion' and 'multidisciplinary working'. This was the starting point for the investigation. The single question that informed the entire investigation was 'how it was possible to do what was done with regards to ADHD in the service in the present moment?' I was aware of tensions in the service regarding ADHD, but yet the procedures for management of the problem appeared to be unquestioningly accepted and enacted. My aim was to attempt to understand what made this possible. As with the chapters above, this chapter is presented in two sections: the first section documents the initial steps of the analysis, highlighting the shifting background within the case notes and meeting minutes that highlight the emergence and influence of the procedures of ADHD that came to form the everyday social practice of diagnosis and treatment. The second section provides an analysis of the discursive background that allowed for the emergence of the procedures and which provided the invisible lines of authority upon which they were legitimated.

The analysis in Chapter 6 offers a conceptualisation of the medication review through the Foucauldian lens of disciplinary power. The chapter highlights the disciplinary process enacted through the 'elements' that formed the medication review by using Foucault's account of panopticism to frame the process as a form hierarchical observation in which normalisation was enacted through discipline. This chapter was made possible through observing ADHD medication reviews, a required procedural component of the diagnostic process. Through these observations, I located a tension between the 'ADHD presentation' represented by formal institutional knowledges and the everyday 'problems' that came to be represented by ADHD. Another tension was the 'treatment' of ADHD. Formal institutional knowledge provides an account of the 'action' of the medication on the source of the 'symptoms', resulting in the behavioural symptoms being 'treated'. The everyday reality of ADHD treatment in the service was at odds with this account, however. This chapter aimed to provide an account of the means by which ADHD continued to be fixed on the young person despite these tensions.

Chapter 7 concludes the investigation by drawing together the elements of the apparatus and situating these within a discussion of the merits of critical ethnographic approach informed by poststructuralist theory. The chapter leaves the investigation open by highlighting the changing nature of the problematisation of young people through the emergence of ASD as the new explanation for problematic behaviour. This new form of problematisation is situated within the elements of the apparatus that allowed for ADHD to emerge.

Summary

The investigation documented in this book relates to the mental health and well-being of children and young people. I am interested in how the knowledges and practices that structure everyday social action relating to mental health and well-being emerge from within an 'apparatus' of interconnected cultural, political, and economic factors. What is offered is a critical ethnographic 'case study', one that connects everyday social actions to a multitude of influencing historic and current social, institutional, political/policy factors and which documents their role in conditioning the possibility of these everyday practices to be possible. The investigation was influenced by and overlaps with an emerging area within global mental health studies. There have been calls within this theoretical domain for approaches that consider cultural, political and economic factors and their interaction with local contextual factors. The approach I adopt is an 'at-home' ethnography, one that utilises the constructs and theoretical approach emerging within the global health movement to explore how contemporary 'problems' have come to be understandable as they are currently known.

Acknowledgements

A lot of people have contributed to this book in various different ways. Without their various contributions, the book would not have happened, and I am hugely grateful to each of them for their support. Firstly, I would like to thank David Fryer and Ravinder Sidhu. Completing the investigation was not straightforward, and I am hugely grateful to you both for your input. I would also like to thank Gordon Tait, Clare O'Farrell, Sue Creagh and Sam Sellar. Each of their reviews were supportive and their feedback helped shape the finished article. I would also like to thank various people who helped smooth the research path in some way – Georgia Laval, Helen Prior, Jacqueline Sproule, Rosemary Wilson, Lorraine Johnston, Doreen Smyth, Joyce Clearie, James and Joanne Boyle, Rose Stambe, Christina Fryer, Matthias Schwannauer and Delwar Hussain. A final thank you must go to the various participants who took part in the investigation.

Chapter 1

Establishing the Research Frame of Reference

Attention deficit hyperactivity disorder (ADHD) is the most extensively studied area of child psychiatry and the most common psychiatric status ascribed to children worldwide. Since first appearing in the *DSM-II* as 'Hyperkinetic Reaction of Childhood', ADHD has undergone multiple changes in nomenclature and nosology, with advocates arguing that this reflects the increasingly sophisticated understanding of the pathophysiology provided by research from neuroimaging studies (see: de Mello et al., 2013); twin studies (see: Kuntsi et al., 2013); adoption studies (see: Harold et al., 2013); and genetic studies (see: Hawi et al., 2013). This evidence is argued to highlight that ADHD is a 'biologically driven, brain-based neuro-developmental disorder', the 'most heritable psychiatric disorder', arises from the 'interplay of environmental risk factors and multiple susceptibility genes' and is 'associated with both structural and functional brain deficits' (see: Faraone et al., 2005; Fischman & Madras, 2005; Seidman, Valera, & Makris, 2005).

The above representation of ADHD is not the only one, however. A brief review of ADHD literature highlights that there are as many critics as there are advocates, a whole range of competing possible causes of the 'symptoms' (see: Armstrong, 1996; Atkinson & Shute, 1999; DuPaul, McGoey, Eckert, & VanBrakle, 2001; Powell & Inglis-Powell, 1999; Shanahan, 2004; Smelter, Rasch, Fleming, Nazos, & Baranowski, 1996; Walker, 2004), as well as multiple alternative explanatory frameworks that would allow for ADHD to be known in a completely different way (see: Baldwin, 2000; Baughman, 2012; Breggin, 2002; Conrad & Schneider, 1980; DeGrandpre, 1999; Ideus, 1995; Prior, 1997; Slee, 1995; Tait, 2006). Even if a brief review were to be confined to only positivist experimental psychiatric and psychological research, there would be as many articles regarding the methodological failings of the 'evidence' as there are articles claiming to provide 'evidence' for ADHD. As means of an example, contrast the questions asked of ADHD neuroimaging studies (see: Castellanos et al., 2002; Fox et al., 1995; Sowell et al., 2003; Walker, 1998), twin studies and adoption studies (see: Joseph, 2000, 2002, 2004, 2006) and genetics studies (see: Arcos-Burgos et al., 2004; Bakker et al., 2003; Bakker et al., 2005; Fisher, Franks, McCracken, & McGough, 2002; Hebebrand et al., 2006; Langley et al., 2004; Mill et al., 2005; Van der Meulen et al., 2005) with the previously mentioned studies in each of these areas regarded as 'evidence' for ADHD.

Given that ADHD has attracted trenchant criticism from many professionals within the field of child and adolescent mental health, as well as commentators and critics outside that field, and that increasingly sophisticated biomedical investigations have failed to produce conclusive evidence of genetic, biological or neurological indicators, why does diagnosis and treatment with stimulant medications continue apace? My aim with this investigation was to consider this question; however, rather than entering the debate for and against ADHD that characterises the mainstream psychological and psychiatric literature, I approach the question from a Foucauldian-inspired sociological perspective. Thus, my approach does not subscribe to modernist assumptions of knowledge as cognitive representation of 'what is the case' in the 'real world' arrived at through positivist-inspired research based on rationality and empiricism. To take this approach would imply that the symptoms of ADHD are naturally occurring phenomena embodied in the sufferer and that the diagnosis is globally and trans-historically applicable, 'out there' independent of its observers and awaiting discovery through objective observation and by experts.

Instead, my position throughout this book assumes infinitely many potential 'reality-versions', each of which promotes the interests of some as opposed to other interest groups. Reality-versions are considered to be constituted at intersections of societal structures and are socially manufactured through legitimation practices into 'knowledges'. The reality-versions that I am interested in are 'psy-complex' reality-versions: 'the heterogeneous knowledges, forms of authority and practical techniques that constitute psychological expertise' (Rose, 1999, p. vii). As such, I do not consider psychological and psychiatric knowledges, such as ADHD, as a description of 'real' phenomena but as constituting them and, in the process of so doing, individualising, psychologising, essentialising and naturalising as inevitable what are contingent socially constituted and so reconstitutable features of particular politico-socio-economic arrangements.

ADHD and the various categories and concepts associated with these psy-complex reality-versions are considered socially sanctioned ways of understanding the world. By producing 'positive knowledges' and 'plausible truth claims' through 'apparent dispassionate expertise', these psy-complex reality-versions have not only made it possible for humans to understand themselves and others in ways that we have come to view as 'psychological' – personality, intelligence, self-esteem, behaviour, etc. – but also made it difficult for humans to be conceived in ways outside of these knowledges. These knowledges have come to enjoy the privileged position of 'truth' within our current historical and cultural period and have provided everyday social practices that reinforce their status as knowledge as well as reinforce the positions of the institutions that enact them. These knowledges, with their implicit norms, regulations, controls and various methods for shaping the individual in the image of the knowledge, have enwrapped us, influencing our thinking and judging, and how we act and interact.

Our current dominant system of truthing structures truth as scientific knowledge; in this sense, ADHD, as an object of psychological and psychiatric knowledge, with its filtering through 'objective' scientific methods and with its enunciation of and enunciation by multiple connected knowledges and practices – such as medical, psychiatric, psychological, educational – and as enacted by various positions of authority – such as psychiatrists, psychologists, teachers – has come to enjoy the privileged status of 'truth'. The rules, according to which the true and the false are separated within the regime of 'truth' of ADHD, evident in the debate between the 'International Consensus Statement on ADHD' (Barkley et al., 2002) and the 'Critique of the International Consensus Statement on ADHD' (Timimi et al., 2004), focus on the rules and procedures that enact 'objectivity' and 'methodological rigour', with conceptualisations that do not attend to these procedural requirements being assigned the status of 'false', or at best 'methodologically flawed'.

Established as truth within our present culture and historical period, ADHD has become embedded within laws, policy, training, 'interventions' and everyday language; these various elements are assembled together into apparatuses which produce, inscribe, examine, debate, analyse, theorise and, with the results, form further elements. It is within these apparatuses of psychological truth that human subjects are 'assembled', constituted as objects of psychological knowledge through various 'techniques of the self' – the various 'ways of thinking, judging and acting upon themselves' (Rose, 1999, p. xvi) articulated by the understandings presented by 'psy' knowledges that enwrap the everyday life of human beings.

'Truthing' ADHD through Psychiatric Research

From its inception as the DSM in 1957, the number of categories of classification has more than tripled, increasing from 112 to 374 in the *DSM-IV-TR*; with the release of the new edition, the *DSM-V*, further concepts and categories have been introduced. ADHD and the multitude of other categories are further divided into 'subtypes' and 'symptomology', allowing for an increasingly nuanced categorisation of human subjects. They have also become embedded in various forms into everyday life, through the internet, through television, through newspapers and magazines, transforming family relations by urging observation ('watchful waiting') (NICE, 2008, p. 15) and readiness to respond to the 'signs of disorder' by placing the child in front of an 'expert'. And with the embedding of ADHD and other categories in policy and guidance, professional relations have also been transformed, with the role of pre-school assistants, classroom assistants and teachers extended into new areas of social management. The techniques for managing difference have also burgeoned with the most common, psychostimulant medication, being the most controversial. However, many further techniques are applied which, although less obvious, are no less insidious. Take any guidance regarding 'treatment' of ADHD or other childhood disorders, and you will have a stepwise approach to the management of difference refracted through a psychiatric lens.

The 'discovery' of ADHD is attributed to George Frederick Still. During the Goulstonian Lectures to the Royal College of Physicians in 1902, descriptions such as 'passionateness', 'spitefulness', 'cruelty', 'jealousy', 'lawlessness', 'immodesty', 'sexual immorality' and 'viciousness' (Still, 1902, p. 1009) were presented as signs of a 'defect of moral control' in children who were deemed too intelligent for the behaviours to be associated with 'disorders of intellect'; the 'defect of moral control' was considered a 'manifestation of some morbid physical condition' (Still, 1902, p. 1165). These descriptions have been presented by mainstream literature as early 'proof' of ADHD before being refined by the 'progress of clinical practice' and 'scientific investigation', both by advocates (see: Barkley, 1990, 1991, 1997) and critics (see: Armstrong, 1995; Breggin, 1998) of ADHD. However, if one were to consider this from a position informed by critical theory and a critical approach to knowledge production, it could be argued that the emergence of this particular object of psychiatric knowledge was not 'discovered' but was constituted through an interconnected nexus of discourses, knowledges, practices and procedures.

As highlighted by Rose (1999), the conditions of possibility for 'psy' knowledges, such as ADHD, to emerge are 'themselves practical and institutional, involving the collection of persons together in particular places, their organisation within particular practices and the grids of perception and judgement that are thrown over conduct and competencies as a consequence [...]; psychological phenomena [...] are thus the outcome of a complex process of production, requiring the alignment of entities, forces, gazes and thought' (p. xv). This is apparent in the series of meetings held between 1948 and 1951 and published in the *Journal of Orthopsychiatry* between 1949 and 1952 (see: Healy, 1949). These publications detail a series of discussions between representatives of the institutions of psychiatry, paediatrics and criminal justice; the focus in the meetings was the applicability of the category of 'psychopath', an object of a moral discourse, when applied to children. It is argued that these meetings paved the way for judgements of morality to slide into obscurity and be replaced solely with a psychiatric judgement; the particular 'alignment of entities, forces, gazes and thought' within these meetings allowed for 'psychiatric' judgements to be 'thrown over the conduct and competencies' of certain groups of children and conditioned the possibility for the emergence of the 'organicity of hyperkinesis', the category from which the modern concept of ADHD emerged.

The 'truthing' of 'hyperkinesis' as 'biological' in origin and as an 'organic child psychiatric disorder' allowed for conduct and competencies that were previously considered a moral concern and for emergence of the rhetorical 'scientific-ness' of ADHD upon which the current battle over truth is fought; once this 'truth' was established, brought into existence, further explored, dissected, analysed and classified, a 'family of descriptions' that formed one version of reality to the exclusion of other versions of reality emerged. And once this 'family of descriptions' took hold, the production of other 'families of descriptions' was closed off as forms of research and investigation followed one path at the expense of others (Rose, 1999, p. xvi). The family of descriptors that currently provide the intelligibility of ADHD is provided by the biomedical discourse, which upturned the psychodynamic discourse that dominated psychiatric knowledge in the *DSM* in which Hyperkinetic Reaction of Childhood first appeared. This shift in 'aetiological focus' emerged from controversies and disputes over the 'truth' between a 'neo-Kraepelinian' paradigm and a 'psychodynamic paradigm' between the second and third editions of the *DSM*; through this confrontation, the concept of 'reactions' associated with the 'psychodynamic paradigm' was replaced by descriptors of the expression of disorders and claims of being 'atheoretical with regard to aetiology' (Klerman, 1978, p. 7). It is through this shift that the principles of the descriptive classification system of Emil Kraepelin and the concept of 'biological aetiology' was reintroduced to psychiatry, which allowed for burgeoning of research in order to establish the biological origins of psychiatric disorders; the 'family of descriptions' and associated practices that have taken hold are connected to the modernist scientific discourse, allowing ADHD to be constituted as a 'biologically driven, brain-based neuro-developmental disorder'.

The Rise of ADHD

Despite the dubious origins of 'scientific-ness' of ADHD and being considered the most controversial child psychiatric disorder, the number of children receiving the diagnosis, and the resulting treatment with stimulant medication, has risen exponentially in recent years. For example, in the UK, a recent report on the safe management of controlled drugs (see: CQC, 2013) highlighted that prescriptions of methylphenidate increased by 236,937 between 2007 and 2012 in National Health Service (NHS) settings in England, an increase of 56% on the 2007 figure. Scotland saw a similar increase in the prescription of methylphenidate. According to the Information Services Division (see: ISD, 2012) of the NHS National Services Scotland, the number of prescriptions of methylphenidate increased from approximately 43 defined daily doses (DDD; per 1,000 of the 0–19 population) to approximately 91 DDD (per 1,000 of the 0–19 population) which, based on the Scottish populations of 0- to 19-year-olds for 2002 (1,210,000) and 2011 (1,172,000) (see: GROS, 2013), was an increase of 54,600 prescriptions (an increase of 105% on the 2002 figure). However, these figures only cover the NHS prescriptions for methylphenidate in England and Scotland; they do not include Northern Ireland and Wales, prescriptions for ADHD drugs other than methylphenidate or private prescriptions. A wider view is provided by the International Narcotics Control Board (see: INCB, 2012); in 2011, the UK had a prescription rate of 0.06 per 1,000 inhabitants per day on all forms of medical amphetamine: at the 2011 census population estimate of 63.2 million, this suggests approximately 3.79 million people were taking a form of medical amphetamine in 2011. This increasing diagnosis and treatment with stimulant medication has also been mirrored in Australia; the number of boys diagnosed increased from 2,200 to 20,800 between 1988 and 1998, with the number of girls diagnosed doubling in the same period. Between 2000 and 2011, prescriptions of stimulant medication increased by 72.9%, making Australia the third-highest prescriber of stimulant medication behind Canada and the USA (see: Graham, 2008; Stephenson, Karanges, & McGregor, 2012).

As highlighted above, ADHD is a global phenomenon; its visibility as explanation for children's behaviour has become more and more prominent, to the exclusion of multiple alternative explanations. It is now common parlance, appearing in newspapers; television shows; radio shows; popular magazines; the internet; on leaflets in GP surgeries and schools and even as an 'app' available for smartphones and tablets.[1] It also appears to be accepted without question by those who are the focus; in my role as a clinical psychologist in a Child and Adolescent Mental Health Service (CAMHS), many of the families I met had requested appointments to discuss whether their son or daughter 'had' ADHD. This was not confined to families with young children: families of teenagers would request appointments, teenagers themselves would request appointments, professionals working with young people would request appointments. What makes this extraordinary is that, whilst ADHD has been available as an explanation in various forms since the 1950s, the rise of the current epidemic of ADHD commenced in the mid-1980s, with a continued rise from its initial emergence. This is evident in the diagnosis rates listed previously, but also highlighted clearly in Figure 1. The chart was constructed using 'Google Books Ngram Viewer', which charts frequency of appearance of specified words in books printed between 1800 and 2008. Figure 2 is focused on the period between 1980 and 2008.

This begs the question: why then? What was significant about this period that allowed for the explanation offered by psychiatric discourse to become so dominant? The answer provided by proponents of ADHD is that the condition is better recognised due to improved training for health and education professionals, improved screening tools, better treatment regimens and the accumulation of knowledge regarding the anatomy and structure of the brain. The implicit proposition here is that lack of awareness, poor training, unprecise screening tools, unwillingness to accept diagnosis due to poor treatment options

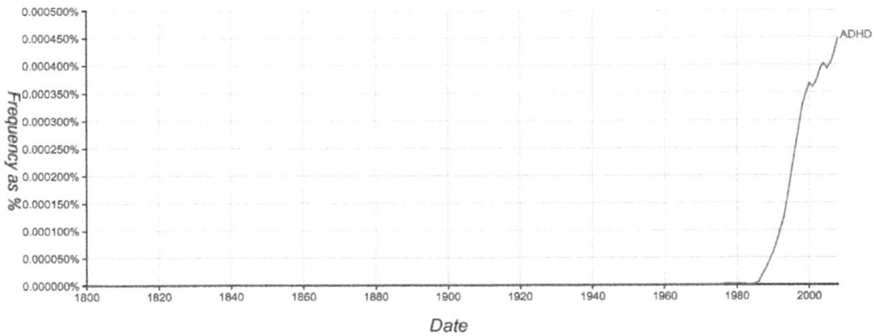

Figure 1: Frequency of Appearance of 'ADHD': 1800–2008.

[1]See: ADHD Psychopharmacology by SoftPsych or *ADDitude Magazine* by New Hope Media.

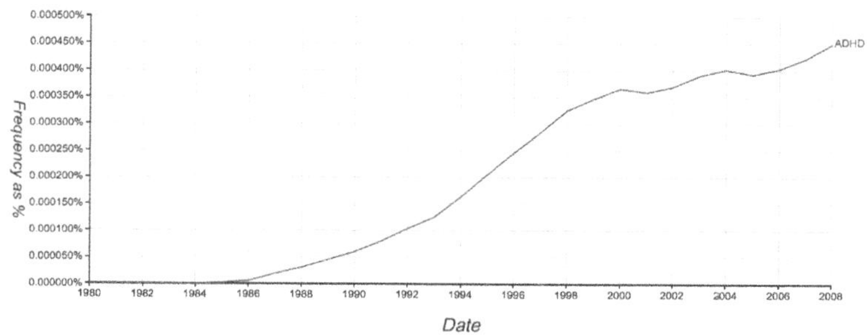

Figure 2: Frequency of Appearance of 'ADHD': 1980–2008.

and lack of knowledge and technology for understanding the origins of the condition have led to an underdiagnoses of the disorder until now. In this book, however, I will offer an alternative account.

Problematising ADHD Diagnoses

The aim of the investigation that I will outline in this book was to question the rising diagnosis rates and the explanations offered for this rise from a Foucauldian-inspired standpoint. The rising diagnosis of ADHD has not gone unquestioned; a recent critique of the expansion of the disorder cited several factors, including a transnational pharmaceutical industry; Western psychiatry; increasing usage of the *DSM* diagnostic criteria; ease of access to online screening checklists; and advocacy groups. I do not dispute these factors as contributing to the rising diagnoses rates, but my point of focus will be different; instead of considering the vehicles that may have allowed for the concept to become more accessible, I aim to consider how the everyday social practice of ADHD has contributed to the burgeoning of usage and, thus, contributed to the rising rates of diagnoses.

To do so, my investigation utilised the concept of problematisation. The concept relates to Foucault's focus on what he called 'the history of thought', which was described as an analysis of the way 'institutions, practices, habits and behaviours become a problem for people who behave in specific sorts of ways, who have certain types of habits, who engage in certain kinds of practices, and who put to work certain types of institutions'. Utilising the concept involves analysis of 'the way an unproblematic field of experience, or set of practices, which were accepted without question, which were familiar and "silent", out of discussion, becomes a problem, raises discussion and debate, incites new reactions, and induces a crisis in previously silent behaviour, habits, practices, and institutions' (Foucault, 2001, p. 74). Thus, my investigation aimed to examine, and call into the question, the gathering together, characterisation, analysis and management of young people through ADHD. To do so, my aim was to examine the interconnected nexus of discourses, power/knowledges, practices and procedures through which young people were constituted as 'having' ADHD.

Discourse, Power and Knowledge

The concept of discourse within Foucault's writing is particularly elusive and difficult to define, mainly due to the different ways in which the concept was used in different stages of his writing; for example, sometimes it was considered to represent a 'general domain of all statements', sometimes it represented an 'individualisable group of statements' and other times it was considered as a 'regulated practice that accounts for a number of statements' (Foucault, 1972, p. 8). For the purposes of this book, discourse is referring to the way it is used in the third definition above: that discourses consist of multiple statements that cohere and produce meaning and effects in the 'real' world. By referring to 'real' in inverted commas, I am not suggesting that reality does not exist, but that the material things to which the categories and concepts that structure our world refer have their meanings inscribed upon them by these categories and concepts and that these categories and concepts gain their specific meaning from the discourse to which they belong. Thus, discourse is considered as a group of statements that belong to a single formation of knowledge and which 'systematically form the objects of which they speak' (Foucault, 1972, p. 54). However, discourses should not be considered as an expression or representation of reality; not only do they produce the objects of which they speak but they constitute particular realities over other realities through defining and establishing what is considered 'truth' at particular historical moments through a 'whole series of particular mechanisms, definable and defined, that seem capable of inducing behaviours or discourses' (Foucault, 1996, p. 394). Thus, the inscription of meaning by discourse constitutes reality, fixing particular understandings and their associated ways for thinking, talking and acting, thereby legitimating the practices and consequences of ordering our world in that particular way.

It is these 'discourse effects', the structuring of the commonly accepted understandings of our world, and the practices and procedures that have been produced in relation to these effects, that were of particular interest to me. As I mentioned earlier, the discourse of ADHD structures commonly accepted understandings about young people, and it has become common practice to problematise young people's behaviour through this particular form of knowledge. As such, various forms of difference are constructed as 'behavioural symptoms' – for example, being 'unable to sustain attention or follow through on instructions', being 'easily distracted', having an 'inability to inhibit response', having an 'excessively high level of activity' – and management of these behavioural symptoms through psychological and psychiatric 'treatments' has exponentially increased as a consequence of these effects. Discourses are able to achieve these effects, to specify 'what is' and 'what is not' in the 'true', through being entwined with power/knowledge. Discourses are historically variable ways of specifying 'truth', with knowledge being produced by effects of power and considered as 'truth'; thus, power functions through discourse, it is constitutive of and is constituted by discourse, thus enabling the fixing of reality through the effects it creates and the 'truths' it establishes. This fixing of reality should not be considered complete, however; we can question our current reality through discourse as it can be both an instrument and an effect of power, but also a hindrance, a starting point for an opposing strategy, as discourse can undermine and expose power, rendering it fragile and making it possible to thwart.

The conception of power offered by Foucault is radically different from previous understandings of power offered within the social sciences; for him, power should be considered as diffuse rather than concentrated, embodied and enacted rather than possessed, enabling rather than purely coercive and as constitutive of subject positions rather than deployed by them. He also did not see knowledge as separate from society or as objective and value free; there is 'not knowledge on one side and society on the other, or science and the state, but only the fundamental forms of knowledge/power' (Foucault, quoted in Sheridan, 1980, p. 283). Thus, for Foucault, knowledge and power are entwined: Knowledge cannot be formed 'without a system of communications, records, accumulation and displacement which is in itself a form of power and which is linked, in its existence and functioning, to the other forms of power' (Foucault, 1997, p. 131). Conversely, it is not possible for power to be exercised 'without the extraction, appropriation, distribution or retention of knowledge' (Foucault, 1997, p. 131).

Foucault's account of discourse and power/knowledge has implications for how we can understand ourselves; if the various knowledges that structure the social world cannot be considered objective truths, but constituted by discourse and power/knowledge, then the ways in which we understand the human subject must be seen as socially constituted and historically and culturally contingent. In this sense, the 'truth' of human subjects presented by psychological knowledge as possessing fixed, authentic characteristics or essences is called into question; people, or rather, the subject positions that people inhabit, are considered the product of power/knowledge, constituted as an object of psychological knowledge through various technologies of power and self. Technologies of power are seen as any assembly of practical rationality governed by a more or less conscious goal, an assemblage of knowledge, instruments, persons, buildings and spaces which act on human conduct from a distance. Technologies of self are considered as the various techniques and strategies that allow individuals to work on themselves – their thoughts, actions, bodies, conduct – in order to self-govern in relation to the norms and orders of particular forms of knowledge.

Power, therefore, is considered to function through the subject positions constituted by discourse, as functioning through diverse social practices, and as productive, as constitutive of the discourses and knowledges that structure our ways of knowing ourselves and others and the subject positions that reinforce these forms of knowledge. However, the particular 'truths' that structure our social world subjugate alternative possible 'truths' by limiting alternative ways of thinking, being and talking through rules that govern what can be considered as true or false knowledge; thus, power should be seen as both a productive and constraining force. In coupling both power and knowledge, Foucault indicates that power and knowledge are co-determinant; power is always bound up with knowledge – they presuppose one another, co-contributing to the production of the subject positions that come to be inscribed upon us and the objects (including alternate subject positions) that we can know about. Thus, power/knowledge provides the conditions of possibility for the social world; power produces the subject positions, the objects, concepts and categories, creating difference in their individual characteristics and relationships by attaching them to specific discourses and knowledges.

Discipline and Governmentality

Foucault's two descriptions of power – disciplinary and governmentality – can be conceptualised as different historical configurations of power/knowledge. The historical configuration of disciplinary power can be conceived of as a 'technology' that gathers information on the body via mechanisms of individualisation and surveillance and which uses this knowledge to induce certain forms of conduct, behaviour, performance and capacities. Through producing certain knowledges of the body, power is able to train the body in certain ways, to perform certain functions and actions; this 'micro-physics of power', as Foucault termed it, 'reaches into the very grain of individuals, touches their bodies and inserts itself into their attitudes and actions, their discourses, learning processes and everyday lives' (1980, p. 39).

The configuration of power termed 'governmentality' can be considered as the present configuration of power (although not superseding disciplinary). By government, Foucault is referring to the techniques and procedures which govern and guide our conduct, 'the broad sense of techniques and procedures for directing human behaviour' (1997, p. 82). In this configuration, power is conceived as operating through specific institutions and their practices in order to exert control, but a control that acts upon subjects through various forms of dominant knowledges and, instead of restricting freedoms, that allows for the incorporation of these into the mechanisms which guide people's behaviour in the social body. Further, the enactment of power does not occur solely within the confines of schools or hospitals, as with disciplinary power (although it continues to be enacted there also), but throughout the social body, through the numerous activities and relationships to which we are located: we, individual human subjects, form this network when we act in the name of a particular knowledge, perform a role for a particular institution or attempt to act upon the actions of others (or ourselves) to influence thinking, judging or acting.

Foucault's concept of discourse and power/knowledge questions are accepted 'truths' – they must be considered as the product of discourse, as embedded in, and produced by, the functioning of systems of power acting through discourse. The truths that structure our understanding of the world do not refer to 'real' facts about the world; they discursively constitute our world, organising knowledge in particular ways, thus providing the intelligible background that governs what can be thought, said or done. Thus, ADHD and the ADHD young person are, therefore, seen as products, constituted though psychological and psychiatric power/knowledge. The ADHD young person is also constituted as 'real' in the day-to-day talk and action of a multitude of professionals and experts as well as by families and young people themselves when they come to know themselves through ADHD knowledge. If we understand forms of knowledge, such as ADHD, as modes of governing the conduct of children and families, as part of the 'myriad methods for shaping human subjects' behaviour and action through the deployment of 'programmes, strategies, techniques' that 'act upon the action of others for certain ends' (Rose, 1999, p. xxi), then ADHD should also be understood as the subjugation of young people 'in the reality of a social practice through mechanisms of power that adhere to a truth' (Foucault, 1997, p. 47). The particular 'truth' is the biomedical 'truth'; the social practices structured and warranted by this, and which subjugate young people, are psychiatric and psychological diagnoses and intervention.

Governmentality and the Apparatus of Truth

In 'two histories of the truth', Foucault (1994b, p. 4) describes two approaches to history: one which was concerned with the development and regulation of forms of scientific knowledge and one which was concerned with human subjects' relation to 'truth'. In this second 'external' history, he draws attention to how subjects' relation to truth is defined by subjectivity, types of knowledge and fields of objects. This relation to 'truth' is considered to be formed by apparatuses of power. Foucault describes the 'apparatus' as 'a thoroughly heterogeneous ensemble consisting of discourses, institutions, architectural forms, regulatory decisions, laws, administrative measures, scientific statements, philosophical, moral, and philanthropic propositions [...], the apparatus itself is the system of relations that can be established between these elements' (1980, p. 194). The concept of the apparatus was utilised to demonstrate the problematisation of 'sexuality' in the *History of Sexuality* and to demonstrate the problematisation of the 'delinquent child' in *Discipline and Punish*. Rose (1999) also made use of the concept in his previously discussed investigation of the development of 'psy' knowledges to highlight the conditions under which their truths, facts and explanations came to be formulated and accepted.

The concept of the apparatus was utilised in this project. In following Foucault, it was my contention that it is within apparatuses of psychological and psychiatric 'truth' that the ADHD child is 'assembled', constituted through discourse, power/knowledge and the practices and procedures that have been constituted by this enmeshment of discourse and power. The most complete description of the apparatus has already been partially described earlier; however, the full statement offers further detail with Foucault adding what he was trying to identify with the apparatus:

> [...] the nature of the connection that can exist between these heterogeneous elements. Thus, a particular discourse can figure at one time as a programme of an institution, and at another it can function as a means of justifying or masking a practice which

> itself remains silent, or as a secondary reinterpretation of this practice, opening out for it a new field of rationality. In short, between these elements, whether discursive or non-discursive, there is a sort of interplay of shifts of positions and modifications of function which can also vary very widely. Thirdly, I understand by the term 'apparatus' a sort of – shall we say – formation which has as its major function at a given historical moment that of responding to an urgent need. The apparatus thus has a dominant strategic function. This may have been, for example, the assimilation of a floating population found to be burdensome for an essentially mercantilist economy: there was a strategic imperative acting here as the matrix for an apparatus which gradually undertook the control or subjection of madness, mental illness and neurosis. (Foucault, 1980a, pp. 195–196)

What is indicated by Foucault is that the apparatus should be considered as a formation of both the 'discursive' and the 'non-discursive'; it is outlined as consisting of multiple heterogeneous elements, one being discourse, but also non-discursive elements, such as architectural forms, regulatory decisions, administrative measures, etc. If one considers discourses as 'practices that systematically form the objects of which they speak' (Foucault, 1972, p. 54) and as one element of the apparatus along with multiple others, discursive and 'non-discursive', Foucault appears to be indicating that the apparatus is a more comprehensive object of study, one that allows for examination of the 'materiality' of discourse. This is also outlined in both of the texts in which he utilises the apparatus as a methodological tool: *Discipline and Punish* (1977) and *The History of Sexuality* (1998b). In *Discipline and Punish*, he highlights the shift in forms of punishment from torture to imprisonment; his description of the 'carceral system' highlights the combining '[...] in a single figure discourses and architectures, coercive regulations and scientific propositions, real social effects and invincible Utopias, programmes for correcting delinquents and mechanisms for that reinforce delinquency' (p. 271). In *The History of Sexuality*, he outlines the movement between two different apparatuses (of kinship and of sexuality) which allowed for the emergence of the technology of sexuality; these two apparatuses are contrasted term by term, outlining 'elements' in each, as well as their strategic function (pp. 106–107). In another text, further clues as to what can be considered 'elements' within an apparatus are offered: 'there is nothing to be gained from describing this autonomous layer of discourse unless one can relate it other layers, practices, institutions, social relations, political relations, and so on. It is the relationship that has always interested me' (Foucault, 2000, p. 284), which further reinforces the notion of the apparatus as the material existence of discourse.

If Foucault's point that the apparatus 'has as its major function at a given historical moment that of responding to an urgent need' is considered alongside the way he utilised the concept in *Discipline and Punish* (1977) and

The History of Sexuality (1998), changing historical relationships between discourses and apparatuses are highlighted as important to consider. In both of these texts, historically specific apparatuses are shown to emerge from previously unrelated apparatuses; this occurred through the production and accommodation of various new and unforeseen elements, generated through the strategic aim in which they were engaged. This is most clearly laid out in *The History of Sexuality* with the emergence of the concept of 'sexuality' from the elements that formed the concept of 'alliance'. Both apparatuses were formations that consisted of the same elements; however, the readjustments of these elements allowed for the strategic objective to shift from the reproduction of 'the interplay of relations' and the maintenance of 'the law that governs them [apparatus of alliance]' to the 'continual extension of areas and forms of control [apparatus of sexuality]' (Foucault, 1998b, p. 117). Through the shifting of the elements that formed the intelligible background of the apparatus of alliance, sexuality emerged, along with a proliferation of associated discourses, institutions, knowledges, practices, norms, rules, relations and techniques of power that maintained it as an object of thought. What was also demonstrated was that the shifting elements were not the result of the agentic action of individuals or powerful institutions, but the chance production of unforeseen effects and the attempts of the apparatus to accommodate these within its various interconnected, heterogeneous, elements. It was through this double process of 'strategic elaboration' and 'functional overdetermination', according to Foucault (1994b, p. 195), that the technology of sexuality was produced and then accommodated as a tool for 'social control and political subjugation' (Foucault, 1998b, p. 123).

The 'management' function of the apparatus is also worth considering in more detail due to its importance in highlighting the empirical relationship that connects the discursive and non-discursive. The strategic aim of the apparatus was clearly outlined by Foucault when he highlighted its role in the governance of a burdensome 'floating population', which posed a problem for the particular economic arrangements at the time. As outlined, the apparatus was the ensemble of elements which mobilised around a particular problem and it was their connection that gave form to the apparatus; the elements were connected by the common purpose they served, the problem or 'urgent need' that was driving the strategic imperative. In effect, the 'problem' at the centre of the apparatus binds the apparatus together, providing the intelligible background from its connected elements. It is this intelligible background that continues to make visible the 'problem' that the apparatus relies upon it for visibility by conditioning what is possible to think, say and do in relation to the 'problem'.

The Apparatus as Analytical Focus

Although the study does not use the term 'apparatus', *Vita: Life in a Zone of Social Abandonment* (Biehl, 2005) adopts a methodological approach that reconnected the various large-scale economic, political and medical reforms and changing family relations that allowed for certain ways of being to be represented as mentally defective and socially unproductive and for abandonment in a 'dump site of human beings' (p. 1) to be considered acceptable. In a 'progressive unravelling' of the story of Catarina, the investigation charts the many domestic and institutional events through which she was rendered mentally defective and socially unproductive. Once rendered defective and unproductive, the shifting, changing forms of judgement that had taken hold in domestic households and medical establishments allowed family, neighbours and medical professionals to consider the act of abandonment in 'zones of social abandonment' as unproblematic and acceptable. Utilising the concept of a 'bureaucratic and domestic machinery [...] that authorises the real' (Biehl, 2005, p. 10), the investigation reconnected the complex network of family, medicine, state and economy in which the abandonment took form, highlighting reality as conditioned by multiple economic, political and social events. It is against this shifting background of intelligibility that judgements of normalcy are made. And it is against this shifting background that the practices and procedures for the management of what falls outside normalcy are constructed. With these shifts and changes, the boundaries of what it is possible to think, say and do are continually changing, determining the life possibilities and conditions of representation that are available for understanding ourselves and others. Throughout the story, Catarina's voice can be seen to be annulled at various life stages by the power relations in which she was caught; her gradual construction as mentally defective and socially unproductive within the foreground of multiple economic, political, social events eventually allowed for the removal of alternative understandings and replacement with an explanation that allowed for abandonment to be seen as unproblematic and acceptable.

As I mentioned above, the concept of the apparatus was not utilised in *Vita*; however, the study utilised the concept of 'invisible machinery' that 'authorised the real'. The concept of the 'invisible machinery' consisted of various, heterogeneous, interconnected parts and, through various shifts and changes, produced unforeseen effects that were then appropriated to extend its reach. Both *The History of Sexuality* and *Vita* also suggest that forms of governance are shaped by 'machinery' or 'apparatuses' – specifically, the way the family and individuals are shaped in accordance with the changing institutional knowledges and practices that are interconnected with elements of other apparatuses. *Vita* is also a 'progressive unravelling' of the 'the knotted reality' of Catarina's condition. By reconstructing this 'machinery', *Vita* highlighted that as the conditions of our lives and the parameters of our local worlds change, our 'most intimate processes: emotion, cognitive style, memory, our deepest sense of self' are remade (Kleinman & Fitz-Henry, 2007, p. 55). Thus, by investigating the concrete constellations in which people's lives are forged and foreclosed, our 'naturalised' understanding of what is socially possible and desirable can be disturbed and enlarged.

Chapter 2: Part 1

Methodological Plan

As was highlighted in the previous chapter, ADHD is a global phenomenon; the rates of diagnoses and treatment with psychostimulant medication have risen exponentially since the 1980s. One could argue that the rise in visibility of the practice has rendered it difficult to conceive of young people outside of its explanation. But given that the explanation has been around in various forms since the 1950s, why did it gain traction at this specific historical and cultural moment? This is the question that led me to conduct this investigation. There have been previous studies that have asked similar questions, such as Conrad and Bergey's (2014) investigation of the expansion and growth of the disorder, but this investigation considered the question from a Foucauldian-inspired standpoint by utilising the methodological concept of the 'apparatus' introduced in the previous chapter.

The main line of enquiry aimed to understand how the 'intelligible background' provided by the apparatus, upon which the everyday thought and action that informed the social practice of diagnosis and treatment of ADHD had come to be formed. By utilising the concept of the apparatus, the answer to the question was to be found in the connections between the elements of the apparatus that provide the field of intelligibility upon which the actions that constitute ADHD take place. Thus, the investigation focused on the everyday thought and action that informed the social practice of ADHD by examining the day-to-day functioning of a United Kingdom National Health Service (NHS) Child and Adolescent Mental Health Service (CAMHS) and the various networks of relations that were involved in the social practice of ADHD across this interconnected system. The aim of focusing on the day-to-day functioning of these institutions was not to reveal who or what was involved but to grasp the 'conditions that make these acceptable at a given moment' (Foucault, 1991, p. 75).

Like Foucault, my hypothesis was that the thought and action that informed the social practice of ADHD was not 'just governed by institutions, prescribed by ideologies, guided by pragmatic circumstances [...] but, up to a point, possess their own specific regularities, logic, strategy, self-evidence, and reason' (Foucault, 1991, p. 75). By approaching the investigation this way, by asking how it became possible for the ideas and actions of ADHD, and the authorities that perform them, to be in place in the present moment, the investigation was interested in the various events and transformations that conditioned the possibility for the current social practice, which constitutes the ADHD young person, to exist. By considering the various events and transformations that allowed the emergence of these social practices, I was also questioning the role of local 'micro-practices' in the emergence and exponential rise of ADHD knowledge and practice more generally. By micro-practices, I am referring to the repetition, on a regular basis, of the myriad interactions that are required to 'enact' particular forms of social relations in which certain realties are maintained.

In this chapter, I attempt to sketch out the methodological plan, but as there is no delineated Foucauldian approach to research, with Foucault himself against prescription, I will not attempt to provide a 'step-by-step' guide for conducting Foucauldian-inspired ethnographic fieldwork. Instead, the remainder of the chapter will be structured around the 'questions' I asked myself when elaborating the concept of the apparatus into the methodological plan that guided my investigation in the field.

What Is an 'Apparatus'?

The most widely circulated statement regarding the apparatus can be found in *Power/Knowledge* (Foucault, 1980b); here, the apparatus is defined as a heterogeneous collection consisting of various elements, including discourses, along with 'the said as much as the unsaid' (p. 194). As highlighted by Peltonen (2004), the multiple elements, both discursive and non-discursive, indicate the apparatus as a comprehensive object of study. Although included as an element, the apparatus moves beyond discourse to include 'other layers', such as 'practices, institutions, social relations, political relations, and so on' (Foucault, 1988a, pp. 284–285). This is also articulated by Rabinow and Rose (2003); the authors endorse the apparatus as 'one of the most powerful conceptual tools introduced by Foucault' (p. 9) as it allowed researchers to move beyond the 'confines of social theory concepts, such as institutions, classes, cultures and ideas, ideologies, beliefs and prejudices'. However, the very term 'apparatus' needs to be considered further due to occluding much of the distinct conceptual linages from the original French *dispositif*.

This is highlighted clearly at the start of the series of lectures on *Psychiatric Power* (2008); the translator notes state that 'there does not seem to be a satisfactory English equivalent for the particular way in which Foucault uses this term to designate a configuration or arrangement of elements and forces, practices and discourses, power and knowledge, that is both *strategic* and *technical*' (Foucault, 1988a, p. xxiii). The comprehensiveness of the concept is articulated in the original French term: *le dispositif* is used to describe an arrangement that has been set up for a specific purpose and which has been designed to have some form of immediate effect. Agamben (2009) offers further examples, highlighting *dispositif* as referring to the part of a legal judgement that contains the decision, or the enacting clause of the law; the way parts of a 'machine' are arranged or, more specifically, the 'diagram' of the arrangement of the components of the machinery; and, in a military context, the set of means arranged according to a plan. This military definition is expanded by Raffnsøe, Gudmand-Høyer and Thaning (2014), who add that the term designates the carrying out of the military plan in time and space, with the particular means available, and with characteristics of the opponent in mind. In addition to these translations, the etymology provided by Raffnsøe et al. is particularly informative: in both French and English, the term derives from the Latin *dispositivus*, which refers to a certain 'something' that has certain 'attributes'. Both the adjective and its substantive form are considered to be derivatives of the Latin verb *dispōnăre*, which 'set in order', 'arrange', 'dispose' or 'form'; the authors indicate that, conceptually, this indicates that some kind of 'activity' must be added to the 'something' and to the 'attributes' of the dispositive.

By considering all of the definitions, the concept can be expanded: it is both a strategic and technical, multi-layered, multi-component machine or collective, constructed with a specific problem in mind, which functions temporally and spatially to achieve resolution to the problem with which it has been constructed to resolve. This complex and layered object of study is clearly articulated by Foucault in *Power/Knowledge* (1980b): he defines the apparatus as a 'thoroughly heterogeneous ensemble of discourses, institutions, architectural forms, regulatory decisions, laws, administrative measures, scientific statements, philosophical, moral and philanthropic propositions – in short, the said as much as the unsaid' (p. 194); but, rather than focusing on these individual elements, we are urged to consider the 'system of relations between these elements' and the 'nature of the connection that can exist between them' (p. 194).

How Does an 'Apparatus' Function?

After expanding the term, the next step was to consider how an apparatus might function; I found the 'strategic function' and 'urgent need' particularly important for developing this understanding. As outlined earlier, the apparatus responds to an urgent need; in Foucault's (1980b) example, this was 'the assimilation of a floating population found to be burdensome for an essentially mercantilist economy' (p. 194). He goes on to state that 'there was a strategic imperative acting here as the matrix for an apparatus which gradually undertook the control or subjection of madness, mental illness and neurosis' (Foucault, 1988a, p. 194). I take the final part of the statement to highlight an important feature of the apparatus: that it transforms 'problems' – in Foucault's account, the 'burdensome floating population' is transformed into 'madness, mental illness and neurosis' – and through the transformation of the problem, the apparatus is transformed. The process of transformation is outlined clearly in *The History of Sexuality* where the 'apparatus of alliance' becomes the 'apparatus of sexuality' due to 'unforeseen effects' that were the outcome of the functioning of the apparatus of alliance achieving its strategic aim. It is through the double process of 'strategic elaboration' and 'functional overdetermination' (1998, p. 195), the chance production unforeseen effects and the accommodation of these within the interconnected elements, that new elements and problems emerge, shifting the focus and strategic aim of the apparatus.

Having elaborated the importance of the 'strategic aim' in developing this element of the apparatus, I then considered the role of the human subject in achieving the strategic aim. For me, the human subject is in a state of constant flux, continually subjectified and objectified by multiple discourses, continually formed and reformed by networks of competing discourses and power relations. I consider the subject as a vehicle for power, with power circulating through the network of relations constructed and installed by the various discourses that form part of the apparatus; thus, the statements that can be made within the social reality of ADHD are determined by the rules of the discourses that function as part of the apparatus. But as outlined above, discourse is just one of an ensemble of heterogeneous elements that interact with each other as part of the apparatus; thus, I consider the statements and actions that are possible within the apparatus to be determined by the rules of discourse, but also by the wider collection of interconnected elements and their interaction with discourse. As I outlined above, the apparatus continually creates and accommodates 'unforeseen effects' which, for me, permeate throughout the network of connections, continually influencing what can be said and done; each statement can, thus, create unforeseen effects that affect change in connected elements, thus allowing for the arrangement of elements to be forever displaced.

I take this continual displacement through the complex network of interactions and influences as allowing for the changing nature of the apparatus. I also consider this to have implications for the human subjects that inhabit the subject positions embedded within the apparatus: statements made and actions performed can have unforeseen effects, thus altering the gird of intelligibility upon which thought and action can take place. It is this continual process that conditions the possibility of what can be: the strategic aim that binds the heterogeneous ensemble of elements organises, temporally and spatially, the pursuit of the strategic aim, but it does not predetermine the results; it disposes in certain ways, but cannot actualise outcomes due to the multiplicity of possibilities that can be elaborated between the elements. For me, this highlights social reality as unfixed and that the current network of connections that form social reality does not necessitate future social reality. In effect, we are always at a frontier of uncharted social reality, and by examining the direction we have come from, it is possible to chart a different direction for how we can proceed.

How to Analyse the Apparatus? How to Analyse 'Social Reality'?

Having outlined the apparatus and considered what it does, the question of how to analyse the apparatus must be approached. As mentioned above, there is not a delineated Foucauldian approach to research that can be followed step by step; the particular approach taken must be informed by the problem being considered and the theoretical underpinning that guides the questioning. The problem I wanted to consider was what made it possible for the social practice that constructs young people as having ADHD to have emerged within the multiplicity of connecting elements of the apparatus. I wanted to reconnect the complex network of power relations, knowledges, discourses, institutions, laws, policies, economic and political events that interacted to allow for the problematisation of young people by psychiatric and psychological knowledges and, thus allow for the emergence of the forms of governance enacted through ADHD knowledge, to emerge as the solution. As previously outlined, the interconnectedness of the elements of the apparatus conditions the possibility for unforeseen effects and their incorporation as new elements; it is this continual displacement that is of interest: it is against this shifting background that the boundaries of what it is possible to think, say and do continually change, thus determining the life chances of the various human subjects that are caught in the network of relations. This interconnectedness is also of interest as it is this that I consider as shaping the focus and function of the apparatus: it is not the agentic action of individuals or powerful institutions that shapes life possibilities but the chance production of unforeseen effects and the attempts of the apparatus to accommodate these effects. For me, this underlines the importance of the ensemble of elements and how they have mutually influenced each other, rather than the statements of individual 'legitimate knowers' or actions of powerful institutions: they 'know what they do; they frequently know why they do what they do; but what they don't know is what what they do does' (Foucault, 1982; cited in Dreyfus & Rabinow, 1982, p. 187). Thus, 'what they do' is important, as is 'what they do does', but it is also important to consider the various elements and events that have allowed for 'what they do' to be able to 'do what it does' at the specific historical juncture at which it 'does what it does': specifically, I see this as indicating that fieldwork should consider the conditions that have allowed for the 'events' that are implicated in the emergence of the social practice of ADHD to be acceptable at the specific moment of their appearance and to understand the interconnected elements that conditioned their possibility.

By events, I am referring to the pluralisation of 'causes' that are implicated in the emergence of specific realities. Like Foucault (1991), and as outlined by Bacchi and Goodwin (2016), I consider events to be both at the level of statements made and also at the level of discourse. The aim of highlighting the interconnectedness of a multiplicity of events is to highlight the 'practices' that gave rise to them, the 'places where what is said and done, rules imposed and reasons given, the planned and taken for granted meet and interconnect' (Foucault, 1991, p. 75). I am using practices in this statement in a different way than when used to refer to social practices, although ultimately both are connected. In referring to social practices, I am referring to the enactment of the procedures that constitute a specific social activity; in the case of my investigation, the procedures of diagnosis and treatment of ADHD. In using practices as the locations where what is said and done, rules imposed and reasons given, the planned and taken for granted meet and interconnect, I am referring to the specifics of 'what was said', 'what was done', 'who was able to say and do those things' and 'what was the wider background in which this occurred'. More specifically, practices in this wider sense refer to the external relations of intelligibility upon which events rely for legitimacy, the connections that make it possible for specific subjects to say and do specific things and for those things to be in the true at that point in time. In this sense, the enactment of the procedures that constitute a specific social activity are contingent upon the wider practices from which they have emerged: the very basis of that what constructs the social activity is contingent upon multiple connections, encounters, supports and blockages within the wider apparatus for their very existence. In this sense, an analytic aim is the reconstruction of the network of connected events, and conditions that gave rise to these, from which the elements that formed and legitimise the social practice of ADHD have emerged.

To aid this analytical aim, the concept of 'problematisation' was particularly important. A number of authors have explicated the concept (Bacchi, 2012; Deacon, 2000; Rabinow & Rose, 2003), with each of these accounts drawn upon in developing the overview specific to this investigation. For Bacchi, the concept of problematisation captures a two-stage process, which seeks to question how and why certain 'things', such as behaviours, groups, phenomena, become a problem, but also how these 'things' are shaped as objects of thought. In the explication, Bacchi refers to Foucault's work on sexuality, highlighting that he was interested in how different eras problematised sexuality, thus making it a particular object for thought in different sites. Thus, in applying this step to the current investigation, I was interested in how young people were constructed as problems and the sites in which this occurred, including the school setting, the health setting, various policies, guidelines and the practices aimed at young people; the aim here was to understand the ways in which young people were constructed, but also the discourse and forms of knowledge that were deployed in the construction of the particular version of young people that was made visible.

By following this approach, my aim was to 'think problematically' about our contemporary social activities, such as the procedures that form the social practice of ADHD, and call them into question by connecting their emergence to earlier problematisations. To do this, Bacchi encourages us to locate 'problematising moments', the times and places where shifts in social reality take place: by locating these moments, we are locating 'crisis moments', moments in which 'givens' become 'questions', where something that was 'previously silent' (Foucault, 2001, p. 74) becomes a problem, thus providing a point of access in the process of emergence of the 'things' that now appear self-evident. However, as both Bacchi and Deacon highlight, these self-evident givens do not become problems due to shifting historical circumstances or because of new objects that didn't previously exist being created by discourse, but because of the 'totality of discursive and non-discursive elements introducing something into the play of true and false', thus constituting it as a particular object of thought. The totality of the discursive and non-discursive, the apparatus, thus means that we cannot see as inevitable that which emerges from these elements as there are a multiplicity of pressures and influences that impact on these outcomes. By locating these problematising moments, we are able to see that what is considered self-evident is in fact the result of the interaction of multiplicity of events at various historical junctures, none of which were necessary or had anything definitive about them; they are the result of 'politics', the multiplicity of strategic connections involved in the construction of the crisis moments at these historical junctures.

Although the location of problematising moments are an important step, further analytical steps are required. As discussed above, these crisis moments highlight our self-evident truths as contingent upon shifts and transformations within the networks of connections between the elements of the apparatus; but what allows for one version of truth to be established over another? To consider this point, I drew upon Bacchi and Bonham's (2014) elaboration of the concept of practices discussed earlier. The authors utilise the concept to describe the operation of knowledge structures, as opposed to linguistic practice, to bridge the symbolic-material distinction that they argue has become lost in much of the work that utilises Foucault's concept of discourse. Foucault uses the concept of discursive practices to describe the groups of relations – the 'body of anonymous, historical rules' – involved in knowledge formation (Foucault, 1972, p. 117); however, these 'rules' are not principles that organise and structure knowledge per se but are formulated as a 'complex group of relations that function as a rule' (Foucault, 1972, p. 74). Foucault offers this distinction with regard to the formation of objects of knowledge when he directs us to 'locate the relations that characterise a discursive practice' (Foucault, 1972, p. 48), in effect the relations that provide visibility and authority. It is through the connection of these relations that knowledge formations are installed and others closed down, creating the intelligible background that allows for certain things said to be considered as 'truth'. From this, it is possible to consider discursive practices as referring to what is said, but also to the rules, or connections of relations, that allow for what is said to be considered as 'truth'. As outlined above, the particular object of interest in this investigation was 'young people', thus the focus was on how they were problematised by these connections and shaped as the target of the specific interventions that these legitimated. It is through this process of problematisation, the *how* of their construction as a problem, that we are able to access the rules that provide the authority for one particular version of reality to be installed as 'real' over all the other multiple possible reality-versions.

A useful starting point for considering the *how* of the construction as a problem is Foucault's archaeological method. Foucault's research approaches are considered to fall into two phases – archaeology and genealogy – with his writings prior to *Discipline and Punish* considered to be his archaeological texts. In practice, the two approaches overlap, with Foucault continuing to use tools from archaeology in his later works. In the archaeological phase, Foucault focused on the system of procedures for the production, regulation and diffusion of statements; the rules that determined which statements are true and which are false in particular historical epochs. Following Foucault's suggestion that his books be used as 'little tool boxes' where 'this sentence or that idea' be used to 'short-circuit, discredit or smash systems of power' (Foucault, 1975b, p. 115), rather than providing a detailed overview of the entirety of the procedures outlined in the text, I will focus on the concepts that were utilised for the investigation: 'the statement', 'enunciative modality' and the 'rules of formation of discursive objects'. I will also draw upon dimensions of analysis outlined by Rose (1999, pp. xi–xii). However, as above, this is not offered as a 'formal analytical grid'; instead, it is provided as an example of some of the critical questions at our disposal for questioning the *how* of construction.

The first of these analytical components is the 'statement', which is considered the 'atom of discourse' (Foucault, 1972, p. 80). For Foucault, statements are not considered to be spoken or written words (although they can be) but as monuments or events, and as having a materiality. By describing statements in this way, Foucault highlights that, out of all the grammatically correct possible statements that could have been, the statement that was made stands out from all other possible statements by virtue of its materiality: it is the statement that *was* made, it was the statement that entered discourse. The special significance of the statement is emphasised if we consider that the production of discourse is 'controlled, selected, organised and redistributed according to a number of procedures whose role it is to avert its powers and its dangers, to master the unpredictable event [unpredictable statement]' (Foucault, 1981, p. 52). This special significance of statements makes them useful for exploring the ways in which they are made visible in the first place: the network of relations that confer authority on them, thus allowing them to take their position within the field of statements that form the objects, subjects, concepts and strategies that constitute bodies of knowledge. However, it must be noted that statements are not solely words spoken or written; they are artefacts that are formed through discourse and knowledge, and which form objects, subjects and places. Thus, statements can be words spoken, words written, diagrams, tools, prescription pads, buildings, building plans, anything that plays a role in installing networks of relations that allow for the constitution of the ADHD young person.

The second analytical component is the 'enunciative function' (Foucault, 1972, p. 209), which refers to the field in which the statement is located and the relations that are 'called up' when true statements are uttered. The enunciative function highlights the 'active nature of the statement: its activation of other statements and its location within specific sets of relations' (Bacchi & Bonham, 2014, p. 184); it is these sets of relations that function together to form the domain of objects, subjects, concepts and strategies that constitute the bodies of knowledge accepted as 'truth'. It is through the enunciative function, the calling up of other 'true' statements, that authority is conferred upon what is said, allowing these statements to be considered true, and prescribing particular 'enunciating' subject positions with important constitutive effects. However, human subjects are not free to say anything they want, when they want and where they like; only certain speakers, saying certain things, from certain places are able to utter 'truth' statements (Foucault, 1972, pp. 50–52). Both of these dimensions to the enunciative modality carry an important analytical weight: both reveal the various elements that confer authority on true statements, such as qualification or professional standing of the 'legitimate knowers' – the *what* that confers authority on the speaker of true statements – but also the institutional sites from where these 'true' statements emerge, which can be considered as further dimension of conferral of legitimacy and authority.

The third analytical component are the 'rules of formation of discursive objects' (Foucault, 1972, pp. 41–42), which are concerned with the way discourse and bodies of knowledge are formed by particular statements and not others, thus making particular thoughts, actions and behaviours possible and others not. The three rules that underpin the formation of objects are 'the surfaces of emergence', 'the authorities of delimitation' and 'the grids of specification' (Foucault, 1972, pp. 41–42) which, when taken together, allow for examination of the means by which certain statements come to construct the objects of particular bodies of knowledge. The first of these rules are the surfaces of emergence, which refer to the social and cultural domains in which the objects appear; the statements a particular object comes to bear are dependent upon the surface on which it appears, thus influencing how the object is constructed. Foucault highlights that the same object will appear differently across different bodies of knowledge; for example, the young person will differ across psychiatric, psychological and educational discourse, and differ again when appearing as an object of political and economic concern. Each of these domains have their own particular conceptual codes, thus determining the particular statements that will come to inscribe themselves upon their object, allowing for consideration of the way the same object – in the case of this project, young people – comes to be constructed and what this allows in terms of action to them and by them.

The second rule is the authorities of delimitation, which is concerned with the authorities that are able to speak of particular objects as objects of certain knowledges. These authorities are recognised through their 'credentials', as having been legitimised by discourse to define and delimit objects of particular bodies of knowledge; in the case of myself as a clinical psychologist, I have satisfied the particular requirements of the institution of clinical psychology through training and regulation by the institutional governing body, thus enabling 'me' as clinical psychologist to speak legitimately and authoritatively about the objects of its knowledge. However, I say 'me' in inverted commas as I am the human subject, the particular individual, that has filled the 'vacant place' (Foucault, 1972, p. 95) of clinical psychologist. I am not the author of the clinical psychologist statements that I utter; I merely occupy a place within the discourse of clinical psychology, which allows for the statements to be considered legitimate and authoritative.

The final rule, the grids of specification, refers to the ways in which particular objects are 'divided, contrasted, related, regrouped, classified, derived from one another as objects' (Foucault, 1972, p. 42) of particular bodies of knowledge. Foucault provides the example of the way psychiatric discourse differentiated its objects from other bodies of knowledge through reference to systems, such as the 'soul', the 'body', the 'life and history of the individual', and 'neuropsychological correlations'. Some of these systems are very much still in place – the life and history of the individual and neuropsychological correlations; however, the young person is also classified, measured and divided against other grids of specification: for example, psychology – executive functioning deficits; educational – learning deficits; economics – unit of economic burden; political – welfare and health-care system drain.

Foucault urges caution with the rules of formation of discursive objects as the application of these rules provides an 'inadequate description': using psychiatric discourse as an example, families or schools, with their system of thresholds for acceptable behaviour, do not merely classify the young person as having difficulties and then present to the psychiatrist for diagnosis of ADHD. The formation of objects is more complex than the straightforward example above; rules of formation can interact in different ways, as well as the rules of formation of different interacting systems of formation crossing over the same object (i.e. in the case of ADHD, both psychiatric and psychological systems commonly interact), allowing for objects to be constructed in different ways, thus expanding the possibilities of what can be said and done with regard to the objects that are formed.

The final analytic components are borrowed from Rose's (1996) outline of the six dimensions through which analysis of the construction of objects can be considered. Rose highlights that the dimensions do not derive a formal methodology but are offered as a means to question the process of construction that takes place for objects to emerge as objects 'in the true'; they are means of questioning the 'connections and relations among diverse elements that have brought our contemporary ways of thinking, judging and acting into being' (p. xii). I will not provide a detailed account of each of the six dimensions, but I will elaborate the two dimensions that I considered important for this investigation: technologies (of power and self) and subjectivities. The first of these technologies, technologies of power, are seen as 'any assembly of practical rationality governed by a more or less conscious goal' and 'an assemblage of knowledge, instruments, persons, buildings and spaces which act on human conduct from a distance' (Foucault, 1972, p. 26). The second, technologies of self, are considered as the various techniques and strategies that allow individuals to work on themselves – their thoughts, actions, bodies, conduct – in order to self-govern in relation to the norms and orders of particular forms of knowledge. As outlined earlier, the subject is considered a product of power/knowledge, constituted as an object of psychological knowledge through various technologies of power and self; if we consider the Foucauldian concept of power as 'a mode of action upon the actions of others for certain ends' (Foucault, 1994a, p. 341) – an action upon the action of others in which others' conduct is influenced by these actions – then technologies of power and self are the various means by which power can constitute a subject of discourse, either by allowing power to work on the individual through the various relations of power in which the individual is caught, or by the application of power to oneself.

Subjectivities, the forms of personhood made available by power/knowledge, are the 'outcome of a complex process of production, requiring the alignment of entities, forces, gazes and thought' (Rose, 1999, p. xv), which involve the 'collection of persons together in particular places, their organisation within particular practices and grids of perception, and judgement that are thrown over conduct and competencies as a consequence' (Rose, 1999, p. xv). We, individual human subjects, form the 'grids of perception', the descriptions that are thrown over conduct and competencies, when we act in the name of a particular knowledge, perform a role for a particular institution or attempt to act upon the actions of others (or ourselves) to influence thinking, judging, or acting.

Methods for the Application of Theory

The above description can be considered an outline of the analytic of power used for this investigation; specifically, the description provided was the analytic procedure used to question how power created effects and outcomes that allowed for the social practice of ADHD to be in place in the present moment. By developing an approach to the analysis of power specifically for this investigation, I was following Foucault's approach of viewing power as situated; his approach to power was not intended to outline a theory of power as a 'context-free, ahistorical, objective description' (Dreyfus & Rabinow, 1982, p. 184). An analytic of power is offered as an opposite to a theory of power – it is offered as a 'grid of analysis' (Dreyfus & Rabinow, 1982, p. 184). In essence, the outline provided was the means employed for considering the cultural practice of ADHD diagnosis and treatment – this follows Foucault's later work focusing on 'rituals of power, centering on certain cultural practices which combine knowledge and power' (Dreyfus & Rabinow, 1982, p. 184) to produce the practices in which the present moment's knowledges and actions that constitute ADHD have emerged. Foucault (1980b) offers a number of methodological precautions for conducting such an analysis, which I have taken into account when developing the methods for the investigation; I will outline these briefly before outlining the procedural aspects of the investigation.

First, investigations should focus on the 'extremities of power', rather than the centralised legitimate forms of power; they should focus on the ultimate destinations, the regional and local forms and institutions, where it 'invests itself in institutions, becomes embodied in techniques, and equips itself with instruments' (Foucault 1980b, p. 96). Second, investigations should focus on the points where power is in direct contact with its object, its field of application – 'where it installs itself and produces its real effects' (Foucault 1980b, p. 97); thus, investigations should aim to investigate how subjects are 'gradually, progressively, really and materially constituted through a multiplicity of organisms, forces, energies, desires' (Foucault 1980b, p. 97). Third and fourth, the investigation must be conducted as an ascending analysis, from the 'infinitesimal mechanisms' to 'see how these mechanisms of power have been – and continue to be – invested, colonised, utilised, involuted, transformed, displaced, extended' (Foucault (1980b, pp. 98–99). A fifth precaution relates to the object of study: investigations should be concerned with the production of methods – tools, procedures, etc. – for the formation of knowledge, as power, 'exercised through these subtle mechanisms, cannot but evolve, organise and put into circulation a knowledge or rather apparatuses of knowledge' (Foucault 1980b, p. 102). A sixth precaution that has guided the procedures for investigation was informed by Raffnsøe et al. (2014): for them, the crucial concern for investigations should be less to 'elucidate theoretically the ontology of a single and independent dispositive [apparatus]', but to 'analyse empirically the way in which several interdependent dispositives [apparatus] revolve around and exercise an influence upon certain social experiences and problematics' (p. 21). For them, and for Foucault, 'abstruse discussions of conceptual and ontological matters' are only worthwhile if they are able to 'serve as torch lights' in 'historically situated as well as diagnostically orientated, empirical and analytical explorations' (p. 21).

Chapter 2: Part 2

Foucauldian-inspired Ethnographic 'Case Study'

The investigation outlined in this book was conducted within an NHS trust that provides health care for residents of three large regions in the central Scotland area. The regions have an approximate population of 300,000, and approximately 70,000 of the population is comprised of children and young people up to the age of 18. The area is comprised of both urban and rural areas with the majority of the population residing in one of the three communities. The region is served by three local government councils, with each providing a number of social and educational services for children: across the three council areas, there are a total of 109 primary schools and 16 secondary schools, three educational psychology services, and three children and families social work services.

The approach to the investigation is considered a Foucauldian-inspired ethnographic 'case study'. As outlined previously, the investigation aimed to understand how the social practice of ADHD diagnosis and treatment came to be possible in the present moment. The starting point of the investigation was observation and audio recording of ADHD clinical appointments and simultaneous analysis of clinical case notes and CAMHS management team meeting minutes. The starting point of observation of clinical appointments allowed me to witness first-hand the procedure of ADHD diagnosis and treatment. By considering the procedure that structured the appointment as a solution to problems that have come to be constructed by psychiatric knowledge, I was able to locate the subject positions legitimated to inscribe ADHD on the behaviour of young people, the means of judgement that aided the process, and the forms of knowledge and discourse deployed in the process.

The clinical appointments I observed were not pre-selected, but were the appointments conducted in the periods of time that I was present in the CAMHS service. As such, the appointments reflected the 'problems' that are considered to be ADHD and the procedural approach deployed in their management. In terms of the procedure for observing the appointments, all participants were consulted about participation in the project by the CAMHS professional conducting the appointment before the appointment took place. If consent was offered, I joined the clinician in collecting the young person and their family from the waiting area, walking with the group through the secure entry, down a hallway to an interview room. As per the ethical clearance requirements for the investigation, I was not to able to speak with the young person of the family or ask questions of the appointment procedure during the session. During the sessions, I was required to sit quietly and observe the appointments without taking notes or engaging with the process. As such, the recorded appointments can be considered as naturalistic a representation of the ADHD diagnostic process as was possible to achieve in a research setting. All recorded appointments were transcribed professionally and, as the investigation was interested in the procedure of the clinical appointment, only verbal communication was transcribed. Each recorded appointment was retained and used in conjunction with the transcribed version when analysing the appointments. In total, I was able to observe ten clinical appointments, with six young people providing consent to record their appointments. The clinical appointments lasted approximately one hour each, providing six hours of recorded material.

The starting point of observation of clinical appointments also allowed for discussion of the project and for consent to be granted to access clinical notes; only participants who had allowed observation of clinical appointments were consulted regarding access to their clinical notes. Although only six young people consented to recording of appointments, all 10 participants provided consent to access their clinical case notes. The combined case notes provided approximately 2,000 pages worth of textual material, with the smallest set of case notes consisting of 24 pages and the largest consisting of 344 pages. Each set of case notes was constituted by three main forms of material: 'official' communications, such as letters to and from referring professionals, letters to and from the wider network of professionals involved in the diagnostic process and various reports from multiple professional groups; handwritten clinical notes documenting the content of individual clinical sessions, telephone calls, and informal communications; and the 'tools' used in the diagnostic process, including questionnaires and psychometric assessments.

The case notes were not processed for the investigation; all case notes were constructed by the same three sections, with each section ordered from oldest communication to most recent. The order of the case notes allowed for a reconstruction of each young person's diagnostic journey, from point of referral to the appointment I witnessed. As with the observation of the clinical appointments, the case notes provided access to the subject positions able to inscribe ADHD on the behaviour of young people, the means of judgement that aided the process, the forms of knowledge and discourse deployed in the process, but also to the wider network of professionals and institutions involved in the problematisation of young people and the various ways in which the problem was constructed. Additionally, the case notes can be considered as a historical record of the practices and procedures of constitution of the ADHD child within the local health service region. The longest time period covered by the case notes was 12 years and the shortest eight months, with case notes reflecting the clinical activity between 2002 and 2008 (six case files) and 2011 and 2012 (two case files) and 2014 and 2015 (two case files). In this sense, the case notes are a historical record of the shifts of power/knowledge that allowed for the 'fixing' of ADHD on the young person; they can be considered as a historical record of the extremities of 'power', highlighting the point where power was in direct contact with its object: the young person.

Another source of data for the investigation were 'minutes' from various team meetings that had taken place in the service over several years. I had not considered this source of material prior to commencing the investigation and only became aware of their existence through asking questions about a change in the diagnostic procedure discovered in the analysis of the case notes. The 'minutes' provided summaries of 342 team meetings that had taken place in the service between 2004 and 2015. The number of meetings that occurred each year varied, with the lowest being 12 meetings (2014) and the highest 56 meetings (2006). The majority of the meetings occurred on a monthly basis across all years (i.e., the Strategic Management Group meeting) with some meetings conducted less frequently (i.e., the Administrative Team meeting appeared to be every six months). The majority of the minutes were three- to four-page summaries of the topics that had been discussed in each meeting and the main responses made with regards to each of the discussion points. However, some minutes were more detailed, with the longest document consisting of 37 pages and providing the background to a meeting where the service structure and specification was designed. Other larger summaries included minutes from annual review days; these meetings occurred annually, were attended by the full-service staff cohort, and would typically last a full day: the average length of minutes from the annual review days was 12 pages. The combined minutes provided approximately 900 pages' worth of textual material.

The minutes were not organised sequentially: all documents were electronic word documents and were stored in a single folder on the administrative team computer in no particular order. On inspection of the material, it was possible to identify the team meeting represented by the minutes and the date it took place, allowing for ordering by team and date. Once ordered by team and date, I was able to hierarchically order the minutes in accordance with the structure of the service, allowing for consideration of the flow of knowledge from the Strategic Management Group meeting through to individual treatment team meetings (ADHD, eating disorder, etc.) or professional group meeting (psychology, psychiatry, nursing, etc.). Once ordered, it was also possible to identify meetings that had emerged in relation to specific problems and the outcome of these meetings; for example, at various time points, minutes from 'steering groups' appeared, tasked with implementing a specific change in practice or developing a new team, with the new team minutes replacing the steering group minutes once implemented.

The analysis of the meeting minutes revealed the various 'problems' the service had to generate solutions to and the impact of these on the day-to-day functioning of the service. This was particularly useful in that I was able to identify and analyse the specific policies that impacted on the service, but also beyond the service relating to the network of connected institutions, allowing for consideration of the role of problems and solutions in shaping thought and action within and across a multiplicity of sites. The highlighted policies were useful in themselves in that these can be considered the 'practical texts' that offer rules, opinion and advice on how professionals are to 'behave' in relation to the specific problems constructed by the policies (Bacchi & Goodwin, 2016;

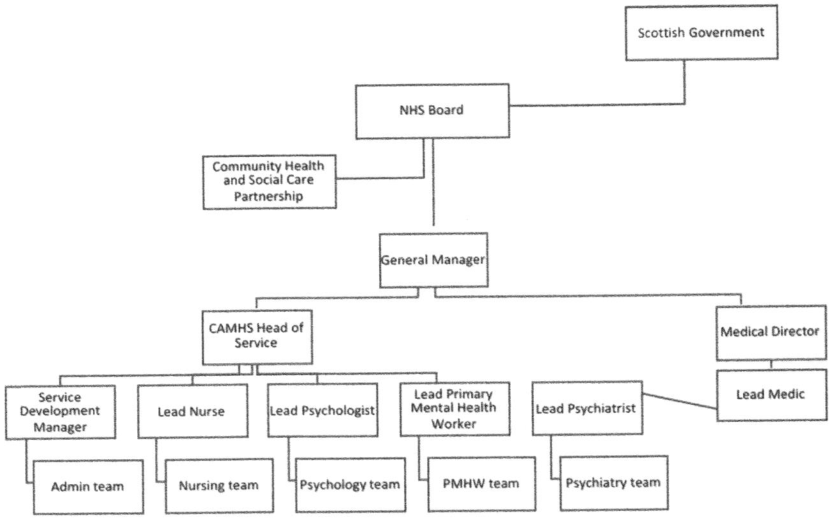

Figure 3: Local NHS and CAMHS Management Structure.

Foucault, 1991b), thus acting as a framework of everyday conduct for those that it targets, both professional and non-professional alike. However, an additional benefit of identifying the specific policies that posed problems and required solutions within CAMHS and the wider institutional network, was that I was able to 'layer' the policies across the discussions that took place in various meetings and then again over individual case notes, allowing for analysis of the ways in which day-to-day thought and action within the service was shaped by and responded to these policies, but also analysis of the emergence of the policies and their constructed problems in relation to wider historical practices, events and relations. Figures 3 and 4 highlight the teams and meetings the minutes represented and the structure of the service, allowing cross-referencing meeting membership with service structure. This was considered important as some team members attended several meetings across the service structure and beyond the service. The meetings beyond the service are not represented in the diagrams as minutes of these meetings were not considered, only references to various outside meetings.

The investigation also made use of interviews with various professionals involved in the wider network identified in the case notes and the sites identified in the minutes. The interviews were not set out in advance; the project was conducted in three six-week periods between 2015 and 2016, with extended periods of time spent in the CAMHS service. The CAMHS professionals were made aware of the project by the head of the service in advance of my presence in the service. The interviews conducted as part of the investigation were follow-up interviews with professionals with whom I had conversed informally during the periods of time spent in the service. They were based on the content of discussions revealing information regarding the emergence of the current social

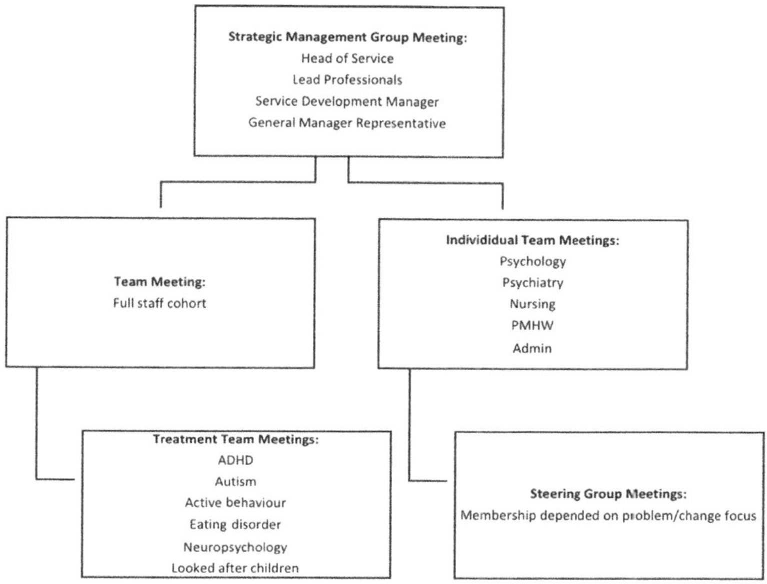

Figure 4: CAMHS Team Meetings with Membership.

practice of ADHD, or questions that arose from observing the clinical appointments or from analysis of documents.

The establishments and educational professionals that took part in the investigation, again, were not predetermined, but were established through the questions that arose from the other sources of the investigation. In this sense, the approach to participation selection for professional interviews can be considered to have followed a 'snowball' approach to selection (see: Faugier & Sargeant, 1997). The general approach is for one participant to provide the details of and organise contact with a second participant, who in turn provides does the same for a third participant, and so on; however, a difference with the approach I utilised was that it was not the participants' connection to a particular group *per se* that was of interest, nor was I interested in what the participants felt or believed about ADHD, but what was said by the participants, the statements they were able to make as part of that group, with the aim of understanding *what* made the *what* that was said legitimate, authoritative, and accepted as 'within the true'.

The interviews conducted during the investigation did not follow a pre-set structure or order of questions. All interviews focused on the same areas: to identify the subject positions able to speak and act in relation to ADHD, what was *said* and *done* by them and what constituted these spoken and enacted manifestations of discourse and knowledge; i.e. what guided their social activity in relation to ADHD diagnosis and treatment? The aim here, as with the case notes, was to investigate the 'extremities of power', the point where power was in direct contact with the young person within educational sites, and to understand what was being deployed in these interactions and the connections that allowed the forms of knowledges and materialisations of knowledge in action to be in the true and deployable in the present moment, i.e. the heterogeneous elements that conditioned their possibility. When possible, the interviews also allowed for questions regarding the connection of educational and health institutions, policies and their role in the social activity of ADHD, and discontinuities in knowledge and practice in both the education and health of children and young people. All interviews were transcribed professionally with only verbal communication being transcribed, as I was interested in the procedure of ADHD diagnosis and treatment, rather than the individuals involved per se – i.e., not what *interviewees* said, but *what* interviewees said, the *things said* and the connections that made the things said, say-able.

A final tool utilised was a library and archive investigation of the historical political and economic background of the locality and the sites that formed the core of the research focus. The procedure that underpinned this element of investigation was adapted from traditional literature review search strategies, making use of the 'Boolean' technique of combining keywords and operators to search archived documents and other textual material. The 'keywords' in this approach, however, were based on 'statements' located through fieldwork, either in conversations with professionals or located in policy. The databases searched included historical, political and economic academic journals, historic governmental policy archives, such the national archives, newspaper archives, and Labour and Conservative political party archives, such as 'The Margaret Thatcher Foundation' and 'The Political Parties and Parliamentary Archives Group'.

Doing 'Critical' Ethnography

The ethnographic approach that guided the investigation drew upon the work of a number of theorists, including Biehl (2005), Madison (2012) and Thomas (1993). The ethnographic approach outlined by Madison is somewhat a rejection of a concrete method in favour of the 'doing of critical ethnography'. In the doing of critical ethnography, critical theory, when used as a mode of interpretation, is considered the method; the critical ethnographer relies on theory to interpret a social action. Thomas further emphasises the requirement for the 'doing' of critical ethnography by highlighting that critical ethnography can be seen as 'the exploration of a common, meaningful cultural world' from which we 'begin to create an understanding of the culture', making use of 'clues, traces, gestures, and scraps of sense' prior to the development of stable interpretations. The collection of these 'synecdoches, or parts of the whole' can then be used to develop an understanding of the whole (p. 15).

Similarly, the study that influenced this project, *Vita* (Biehl, 2005), employed conventional ethnographic tools for different tasks at different points as the study unfolded. As for critical theory being the method, Biehl states that he 'reads and borrows from the language of many books to understand the world he is investigating' and takes these understandings into the field 'where their propositions might not always work that well but are nonetheless helpful in generating figures of thought' (Biehl, 2005, p. 14). *Vita* also emphasised critical analytic tasks that cross-over with the approach adopted for this investigation; specifically, 'make visible the intermingling of colloquial practices and relations, institutional histories, and discursive structures' (Biehl, 2005, p. 23), 'trace the complex network' in which 'pathology' takes form, and explore the ways communities, families, personal lives and inner worlds are 'remade under the impress of economic pressures' (Biehl, 2005, p. 23) by scrutinising the 'bureaucratic and domestic machinery of inscriptions and invisibility that authorises the real' (Biehl, 2005, p. 10).

By employing ethnography as a 'way of looking' (Wolcott, 1999, p. 41), as the doing of the critical theory outlined in first part of this chapter, my approach aimed to reconnect the various elements of the 'apparatus' of ADHD, the heterogeneous elements that conditioned the possibility for the emergence of the everyday practice of ADHD, using the ethnographic tools of observation, document analysis and interview in an iterative and retroductive manner. By approaching the investigation in this way, my aim was not to investigate ADHD as a 'real' condition, but to investigate the conditions fundamental to its existence and usage within the social practice of diagnosis and treatment of the locality in which the investigation was conducted. In this sense, the project can be considered theory-driven research, with the account of the apparatus the a priori knowledge that guided the investigation. It was this a priori knowledge that acted as the means of discovering and questioning the 'conditions', the circumstances without which something cannot exist; in this case, the conditions upon which the social practice of ADHD diagnosis and treatment was produced, sustained and modified locally.

More specifically, the project used a critical theory-driven ethnographic approach to investigate how 'governmental practices', understood expansively as the 'heterogeneous strategic relations and practices that shape who we are and how we are to live' (Bacchi & Goodwin, 2016, p. 14), produced 'problems', thus legitimating the means for solving these problems, and how this process was implicated in the production of ADHD locally as a solution. By problems, I am following Bacchi and Goodwin in viewing 'problems' not as a something that exist in a material sense, but as something that has 'come to be', that has been constructed, through the interaction of multiple knowledges, practices, and events. The approach, thus, investigate how certain problems 'came to be' problems in order to reveal their ontological politics, the various interconnected elements that constructed these 'things' as problems allowing them to become a target for intervention.

By investigating 'problems' and 'solutions', this investigation adopted a similar approach to that of Bacchi and Goodwin (2016) and Rose (2000). For Bacchi and Goodwin, a key analytic task involves 'teasing out the conceptual premises underpinning problem representations, tracing their genealogy, reflecting on the practices that sustain them and considering their effects' (p. 17). Similarly, Rose urges for an analytical focus on 'answers' to 'arguments', arguing that their very status as answers is entirely dependent upon the questioning of a something that requires to be answered. The presence of answers and question indicates problematising activity which, through reconstruction, allows for the interrogation of the networks of connections that provide the answers with their intelligibility. Through locating a problem and how it is represented and solved, the aim is to work backwards, or outwards from the problem, and to critically examine the network of connections upon which they are based: the assumptions, familiar notions and unexamined ways of thinking upon which the problem and solution rest.

This backwards/outwards reading was a key task as this allowed for examination of the history of things assumed to be natural, the reasons behind their way of being, their material effects, and what they allowed to follow. A further key task made possible by a consideration of problems and solutions was the locating of unforeseen effects and their accommodation within the interconnected elements of the apparatus. As outlined earlier, the strategic aim that connects the heterogeneous ensemble of elements of the apparatus, due to the multiplicity of possibilities that can be elaborated between them, does not predetermine the results, it can only dispose in certain ways, thus allowing for the production of unintended effects. The incorporation of these unintended effects creates continual displacement, creating changes in the problems represented and solutions proposed, allowing for a critical examination of 'what follows from the effects'; i.e. the historical shifts and changes of the interconnected network of elements that constitute the apparatus.

As mentioned earlier, the starting point for the investigation was observation of the clinical appointments and analysis of clinical case notes. Through discussing a discontinuity in practice visible in the case notes, I discovered the meeting minutes, which provided insights into the various pressures within the CAMHS service and across the connected network of institutions, as well as a number of specific policies that placed procedural requirements on the service and beyond. By 'layering' these sources of material, from individual clinical appointment to policy and political and economic archived material, I was able to reconnect the discursive field in which the current ADHD practice emerged, allowing for an examination of what was possible to say and do about the problem of young people within education and health sites, but also consider discontinuities in how problems of young people were constructed across time and place, what was legitimated as solution by these construction, what effects were created, and what followed from these effects.

Through 'layering', I was able to read both horizontally and vertically from the clinical appointment and through case notes, meeting minutes, and policies, and use the analytical components described earlier to locate, track and document the changing discursive background: who was speaking, what was said, what was done, what knowledges and technologies were put to work, how this changed across time and place, who appeared and disappeared, what appeared and disappeared. The aim was a develop a theoretical redescription of the rise of ADHD diagnosis and treatment locally, one that mapped and made visible the multiplicity of heterogeneous elements implicated the construction of young people as particular types of problems and to provide a genealogical account of the emergence of a local practice of ADHD diagnosis and treatment from within this complex network.

Applying Rhizomatic Logic/Offering a Topological Account

In the translator's foreword of the second volume of *A Thousand Plateaus: Capitalism and Schizophrenia*, the question of whether the book can be 'played' (Deleuze & Guattari, 1987, p. xiii) is asked and discussed. The point made is that we should approach the book like the playing of a record, with the book offered as an 'open system', where the reader could start at any chapter and read in any order, generating different meanings depending on the order in which reading occurred (p. iv). Underpinning *A Thousand Plateaus* is the concept of the rhizome, which has 'no beginning or end; it is always in the middle, between things, interbeing, intermezzo' (p. 27), allowing for movement from the 'middle, through the middle, coming and going rather than starting and finishing' (pp. 27–28). I found the concept of the rhizome useful for resolving a problem I had in approaching this project; the linear logic inherent in writing did not match the approach to reading and thinking that was employed, and when attempting to write, I found myself restricted by the linearity in that it created a sense of cause and effect that I did not consider an element of the apparatus.

Thus, by employing a rhizomatic logic, by moving horizontally and vertically through the different texts – from case notes to meeting minutes, back to case notes, over to a particular policy, over to an interview, back to a policy – like St Pierre (1997, p. 179), I was able to avoid the 'ruthlessly linear nature of the narrative of knowledge production'. The 'lateral' logic of a rhizomatic approach allowed for a dynamic, flexible approach that captured the complexity, heterogeneity, and ever-changing 'becoming', rather than a fixed and finished 'being', created through the interaction of the elements of the apparatus. The approach also helped guide my approach to writing; rather than following a conventional linear approach, I found writing the 'node' or 'element' of the apparatus that emerged as most prominent through the rhizomatic logic beneficial as it resulted in a process of movement between and within sections. By employing this approach, like a rhizome itself, each of the sections became detachable, reversible, and the focus of constant modification, being written, rewritten, placed and replaced depending on the reading of, and connections being made within, the different texts.

The Apparatus as a Topology: A System of 'Correlations'

This project is, ultimately, attempting to account for a multiplicity of transformations and effects, occurring within and across a nexus of intersecting elements, which allowed for the problematisation of young people in certain ways, and the eventual emergence of the local social practice of ADHD diagnosis and treatment to be in place. The 'final' description should not be considered as fixed and complete, however; but as partial, as incomplete and unfixed, as a snapshot of a moving process that commenced before and continues after the artificial boundary imposed by my investigation. But unlike *A Thousand Plateaus*, the final description cannot be considered an 'open system', where chapters can be read in any order, as the requirement to frame the project and outline the methods imposes a starting point; as such, the problem of linearity remains present within the writing to some degree because of this imposition. To challenge this, the concept of topology is useful, particularly the account provided by Collier (2009). In this account, the conditions of possibility for what is thinkable, doable and sayable are not found in stable systems of discourse or power/knowledge regimes, but amid the movement and upheaval of problematisation, within the 'patterns of correlation' through which heterogeneous elements are configured and reconfigured. A topological account aims to describe heterogeneous spaces, but also the dynamic process through which the elements of the space are taken up and redeployed, and through which new combinations of elements are shaped. A topological account is not a 'before and after' picture, but an account of how various elements and forms of power have become combined in 'complex edifices', or 'systems of correlation', allowing for certain activities to be thinkable and practicable.

In this sense, beyond the account of the methods used for the project, each section is offered as a point of intersection, where a multiplicity of connecting knowledges, discourses, practices and events exist. The multiplicity of connections is not the result a linear flow of truth or knowledge development, but the result of the effects created through these connections, and the multitude of eventualities that emerged from the conditions created. It was this understanding that allowed me to 'see' the apparatus: the apparatus emerged through small discoveries of elements and connections, which became meaningful through further small discoveries, made possible through the rhizomatic logic described earlier. Through following 'lines of flight' from one site to another, I was able to consider elements as discursive plateaus, as apparatuses of meaning, as systems of correlations that did not stand alone but which informed each other and which could only make sense when considered within and against each other. Through this process, both the elements and the apparatus emerged in tandem: the elements only becoming meaningful within the whole system of correlations and whole systems of correlations only becoming meaningful through the individual elements; what this conveys is that a certain distance must be employed when considering the following sections, one that allows for the individual elements and the whole system of correlations to exist and inform each other. The account provided is not a 'before and after' picture, nor an account of cause and effect; it is an attempt to describe a moving process, one that continues to move beyond the boundaries of this account.

Chapter 3: Part 1

Deindustrialisation, Post-industrialisation and the Changing Requirements of the 'Young' Citizen

The following chapter provides an overview of the changing politico-economic background of the region and requirements of the young person that emerged from within this process. The chapter documents the decline of industry in the region, connecting this with the enactment of 'deindustrialisation' and its role in conditioning the current levels of poverty and disadvantage in the region. The aim of the chapter was to reconnect wider historical political and economic events long silenced by a changing discursive background. What is documented are considered elements without which the current reality of ADHD locally may not have emerged. The elements described are not offered in a linear cause and effect manner, but as correlating events that conditioned the possibility for the effects that followed. These elements are connected to the present in that they are considered part of moving and changing apparatus from which the local procedures of ADHD of gained legitimacy.

The particular focus of this chapter was made possible by the analysis in the following chapter – specifically, the emergence of the requirement for schools to contribute to 'eliminating' disadvantage and poverty. The local disadvantage and poverty was prominent throughout my discussions with educational professionals. Its visibility took the form of accounts of its impact on the civic fabric of the region but also 'on' the behaviour of local children. I previously worked in the region for several years and had only known inequality and disadvantage; I had noticed architecture indicating an industrial past, but had not connected this to prosperity due to the prominence of disadvantage. My previous unquestioning acceptance of this disadvantage was disrupted by a conversation with an educational professional, which illuminated a requirement to question and understand what had happened locally to move the region from a position of relative prosperity to high levels of disadvantage and poverty.

The conversation with the educational professional was my first meeting with them. As a starting point in our discussion, they provided a brief social history of the region, highlighting that the building we were sat in was once part of a thriving milling community that provided employment to school leavers from the area:

> The building we're in at the moment was a mill and as I said to you one of the guidance teachers who works in our Academy at the moment, he remembers the managers, the foremen and whatever, of this mill coming in – you know – to the fourth years and saying right, who wants jobs? Right you, you, you – turn up at the office on Monday and sign up.

Milling was not the only thriving local industrial area, however, with agriculture, mining, shipbuilding, wool and textiles, glassmaking, weaving, brewing, malt whiskey distilling and barrel cooperage all present in the area until relatively recently. Historically, the prosperity of the local region was recognised as, in proportion to its size, being one of the wealthiest counties in Scotland. In the present, however, whilst including communities of outstanding prosperity, the region has neighbourhoods whose health, income and employment standards sit with the poorest in Scotland. In a Scotland-wide context, the region has the fifth highest share of population living in the 15% most deprived areas and a higher percentage of young people living in the most deprived areas in Scotland compared to the Scottish average (see: Office of National Statistics, 2011; Scottish Public Health Observatory, 2008).

The recollection in the conversation above regarding the ease with which school pupils could leave school and take up employment is borne out by economic data from the time; at the end of the 1960s, the region had an unemployment rate of approximately 1.5% of the local population throughout the 1950s and 1960s, lower than the upper limit of 3% that defined 'full employment' within Keynesian economics that dominated post-war British social organisation. However, by the mid-to-late 1980s, unemployment had increased to 18.4%, with 37% of jobs in the manufacturing industry, the industries dominant in the region, lost between 1971 and 1981. Unemployment in the region exponentially rose in a relatively short period: by 1979, unemployment had doubled, and by 1983 it had doubled again, with continued increases from 1983 onwards, reaching 18.4% of the population by 1986, a sixfold increase over a period of 20 years. The labour market was particularly problematic for young people, with over a third of males aged 18 to 24 experiencing unemployment within the previous 12 months, double the figure for older males; by 1985, 16% of males and 24% of females who were out of work were under the age of 20. The impact of the changing labour market on youth employment is most clearly documented by considering the destinations of school leavers: around 75% of pupils leaving school in 1978 had gained employment by the following year, with the proportion in youth training schemes (YTS) less than 8%. However, by 1985, the percentage of school leavers in employment by the following year had dropped below 30%, with the proportion in in YTS rising to nearly 40% (see: Fraser & Sinfield, 1987).

Explaining (Away) the Changing Fortunes of the Region

There are various differing accounts for the increasing unemployment rate in Scotland over this period. One such explanation was present in one of the conversations I had with a local educational professional – that industry was too expensive and not competitive in the newly emerging global economy:

> Along with lots of places in the 1980s, the government policy was that because these were big booted industries and they were expensive to run and there were cheaper imports coming in from other parts of the world so – you know – especially since a lot of them are state funded, these industries like the steel industry, the coal industry et cetera, et cetera – I'm guessing the government policy was this is not financially viable in the long run. Yes, it employs our citizens but actually we can't afford it. And a lot of these things were closed down.

The account above contains statements that can be connected to the historical problematisation of industry which continues in present-day accounts of the exponential rise in unemployment occurring in the 1980s: specifically, that the decline of industry was the result of an unproductive and unskilled workforce, inflated wages and the long-term failure of industry to keep up with the technological advances of international competitors. This account, however, can be seen to silence various effects of the enactment of politico-economic rationalities associated with the 'New Right' and their role in the conditions of the present.

These political and economic theories, an amalgam of contradictory strands of liberal and conservative political and economic rationalities most widely known as neoliberalism, emphasise the efficiency of market competition over other forms of societal administration, prioritise the capacity of individuals in determining economic outcomes through rational choice making and problematise all forms of regulation as reducing the efficiency of the 'natural' function of the free market to regulate society. Despite only gaining prominence in the 1970s and 1980s, these rationalities have become so familiar that it is hard to imagine a background structured differently. And it is this familiarity that allows for the inevitability contained in the statement above – 'if businesses are not financially viable, they are closed down, even it employs our citizens' – allowing for the uncomplicated acceptance of the making redundant of large numbers of individuals. This is to not say that this was the position of the professional I spoke with, but the regular acceptance and use of the explanation continue to silence a historical period when closing down industry and making citizens unemployed was not the norm. And through this silencing, the social and political upheaval associated with this shifting politico-economic background, and their role at present, also remains hidden.

This shifting background is particularly important to this investigation as it played a fundamental role in shaping the understanding we have of 'young people', what we expect from them, what we do to achieve this and what we do when this is not achieved. The shifting background is important to this investigation in other ways too, in that a number of artefacts from this period of social and political upheaval, particularly youth unemployment and reforms to education and health services, played and continue to play an important role in conditioning our present, but they have disappeared from our accounts of the present, allowing for uncomplicated acceptance of the here and now. This investigation attempts to bring them back out, 'unsilence' them and place them in the foreground, allowing examination of their role in conditioning the possibility for the social practice of ADHD.

Troubling the Explanation: Making Visible 'New Right' Rationalities

The various discursive strands constituting the political and economic rationalities of the 'New Right' are widely accepted to have gained dominance from the 1980s onwards. The discourses had been in circulation prior to the 1980s, however, appearing in various political discourses and movements, such as 'Powellism' (see: Nairn, 1970), the 'Selsdon' agenda (see: Barry, 2005), and the 'Ridley report' (see: Gamble, 1988), but the interaction of various political and economic events in the 1970s and 1980s allowed the statements to coalesce around the problematisation of the prevailing social democratic organisation of society. Prior to this historical juncture, the UK was considered a dominant and prosperous industrial nation, attributable to a colonial past of forceful extraction of raw materials for the manufacturing process and a system of economic relations through enforced free trade. After the Second World War, the international economy was reordered in accordance with the Bretton Woods agreement and the Marshall plan, with established economic trading links reconfigured to create a system of trade between advanced industrial societies at the expense of the previous colonial networks. This newly constructed network of interconnections created interdependence in the production and consumption and the import and export of manufactured goods within and across multiple advanced nation states, but also the potential for domestic economic vulnerability through fluctuations and crisis in any of the interconnected nations.

The UK was considered to have been particularly vulnerable to these fluctuations through attempts to maintain its colonial past. High levels of government and private investment in colonial outposts are considered to have underpinned recurring government balance of payment crisis and a lack of investment in domestic industry and economy, which were disguised by post-war economic expansion. The interconnected economic system created new requirements for growth in production and profit across the network, with measures for its calculability and comparability across the network, allowing for economic performance, growth and productivity to emerge as political arguments in the late 1960s and 1970s. A major economic event to impact on the newly constructed network of nations, the oil crisis in 1973, can be seen to have created the conditions for the first appearance of these political arguments, allowing for the impact of the

UKs colonial past on its domestic economy to be reconstituted as an inefficiency of the labour force and an underperformance of industry and for 'deindustrialisation' to emerge as a solution to the 'problem'. The effects from this solution are well documented: from a peak in 1966, employment in manufacturing was 8.4 million; by 1983 this had reduced to 5.5 million, representing a 34.5% fall in 17 years, with half – 1.5 million jobs – lost between 1979 and 1983. In Scotland, by 1979, one-third of the population worked in industry; by 1984, it was less than one-quarter. Scotland's manufacturing was reduced by approximately 30% with the three traditional mass employment sectors – shipbuilding, steel manufacturing and coal mining – all but disappearing (see: Naysmith, 2013; Rose, Vogler, Marshall, & Newby, 1984; Smith, 1988).

The Requirements of 'New' Citizen of the Post-industrial Society

Another often-deployed explanation for deindustrialisation is that the economy required 'modernising' and that deindustrialisation was a necessary first step in this process. The explanation can be considered to be informed by economic and political discourse dominant in the 1950s and 1960s which constructed advanced industrial societies as destined to move from the production and consumption of goods to a post-industrial society underpinned by the 'centrality of theoretical knowledge as the source of innovation and policy formation' (Bell, 1976, p. 12). In this new societal order, industry would be a relic of the machine age and abandoned to the 'lesser' economies of the world with the more 'advanced' economies underpinned by technology, finance, entertainment/service and the production of knowledge and skills.

Employment in this new societal organisation would require flexibility, technical skills and professional qualifications. The requirement for manual labour, physical exertion and the production and distribution of physical objects would be reduced, and employees would gain greater freedoms and control over their conditions of work. The shift to the post-industrial society would occur 'naturally' as the country became richer, with the 'third sector' expanding as industry shed labour and eventually overtaking industry as the main employer of the citizen. The requirements of the citizen in this new societal order would be different than the previous industrial society, with individual freedom, personal choice, self-fulfilment and initiative separating the post-industrial citizen from the passive and state-dependent industrial society citizen. The new citizen would display self-interest, individual moral responsibility and the exercise of personal choice within a free market place resulting in self-enhancement and well-being and a reduction in the requirement for state-provided welfare services.

The material effects of 'modernisation' through deindustrialisation were quite different, however: the discourse of the post-industrial society constructs the shift from industrial to post-industrial as 'naturally' occurring, one that occurs as society grows richer and as employment moves from industry to the third sector. In 'reality', however, the shift from manufacturing to the third sector did not happen; between 1979 and 1983, in the UK, manufacturing output was reduced by approximately 28%, with the reduction in Scotland higher due to a higher concentration of heavy industry and manufacturing. In 1979, one-third of Scots worked in industry; by 1984 it was less than one-quarter, with manufacturing reduced by approximately 30%. Over the same period, against losses of almost a quarter of a million manufacturing jobs in Scotland, employment in the service sector increased by 30,000 (see: Collins & McCartney, 2011; Leys, 1985; Smith, 1988).

Rather than being presented as a problem of the application of New Right politico-economic rationalities, however, the solution to high unemployment levels was to reform the social security apparatus according to the same New Right politico-economic rationalities. The various 'reforms' reduced the financial assistance available and created a requirement for those in receipt of welfare to have their 'need' reviewed on a regular basis, conditioning a shift in the welfare apparatus from one based on universality and welfare to one based on conditionality and workfare. This new welfare apparatus, rather than functioning as a safety net, would function as a technology for disciplining the newly redundant industrial workforce through regimes of assessment of job seeking and a reduction in the amount of financial assistance available. Two reforms specific to young people and relevant to this investigation include the ending of entitlement for school leavers under 18 years old and a reduction of school leaver entitlement for 18-year-old school leavers, both of which will be touched upon later in the chapter.

An unforeseen effect of the New Right rationalities and reforms was increasing unemployment, increasing social inequality, rising levels of social unrest and a resulting impact on social cohesion. Through the slow eroding of the social democratic politico-economic concepts of social integration, solidarity and collectivism and replacement by the New Right concepts of individual responsibility and self-interest, the obligations of the state to the citizen and from individual citizen to the state were disrupted and displaced. As before, however, these effects were constructed not as problems of New Right politico-economic but as the result of passivity and dependency of the social democratic citizen. Against this problematisation, the 'active' citizen, and the 'enterprising culture' in which they would flourish can be considered to have emerged as a solution. The 'active' citizen can be considered as an attempt to counterpose collectivist welfare approaches and the 'dependency' of the social democratic citizen whilst reintroducing social obligations. This new form of citizenry would be both individually and socially responsible for him/herself, their family and others through forms of voluntarism, with state support constructed as a last resort.

Fabricating the Young Active Citizen: The Apparatus of Education

The shifting apparatus of social security can be considered as having the image of the active citizen as its aim. The new regime of reduced financial support, surveillance and disciplinary procedures can be seen as a technology for governing those in receipt of welfare through inducing poverty, with the aim of encouraging movement towards employment in the newly emerging third sector (despite there not being one). Alongside targeting the newly redundant industrial workforce, the specific welfare 'reforms' targeting the young person can also be considered as technologies of discipline. However, both 'reforms' – removing entitlement for school leavers under 18 and reducing entitlement for 18-year-old school leavers – can be seen to connect to a wider approach of governance of the young person involving the apparatus of education. This is visible in the gradual emergence, within the apparatus of education, of discourses and technologies aimed at shaping the young person as a future adult/worker, which are clearly visible in the 'National Curriculum' introduced by the 1988 Education Reform Act. The aim of this new centrally directed national curriculum was to extend educational reach into new domains of the young person – including spiritual, moral, cultural – and for these domains to be utilised in preparing the young person for the 'opportunities, responsibilities and experiences of adult life' (Her Majesty's Government, 1990, p. 3). These new aims would be achieved through additional reforms codified by the act, including instruction in new technological and vocational knowledges and the introduction of regimes of multiple testing, allowing for surveillance, measurement and comparison over time.

The discourse of active citizens can be seen to emerge within the educational apparatus in the 1990s, as evident in the intersecting policy agendas of *Encouraging Citizenship* and *Curriculum Guidance 8: Education for Citizenship*. Both policy agendas attempt to construct a 'consensus view of citizenship'; minimise the contested nature of the concept; and position the pupil, the teacher, the parent and the newly constructed position of school governor as a partnership that would shape the participative and active young citizens of the future. The policy agendas can also be seen as the reconstitution of educational practice as a technology of governance, one that would develop in the young person the 'knowledge, skills and attitudes necessary for exploring, making informed decisions about and exercising responsibilities and rights in a democratic society' (National Curriculum Council, 1990, p. 2), 'establish the importance of positive, participative citizenship' and 'help pupils to acquire and understand the information on which to base the development of their skills, values and attitudes towards citizenship' (National Curriculum Council, 1990, p. 5). This new form of citizenship placed at the centre of the apparatus of education was one based on 'values' that exemplified the 'civilised society'. The overarching emphasis of this new focus, however, was on the responsibilities and obligations of the future citizen to the state, rather than rights of the future citizen of the state. The active citizen would be responsible for themselves, responsible for their development and role within the new emerging post-industrial society, and responsible for others through voluntarism, with the state functioning as night-watchman, as umpire in the post-industrial society governed through free market principles.

A further important shift within the apparatus of education that can be considered a solution to the effects of the enactment of the post-industrial society was the emergence of the requirement for vocational training, as evident across several intersecting policy agendas, including 'A New Training Initiative: A Programme for Action', 'A New Training Initiative: A Consultative

Document', 'Better Schools and Working Together: Education and Training'. The problem constructed across these agendas is a lack of workforce available to meet the new demands of the post-industrial society: the emerging new markets of the post-industrial society are constructed as requiring the adoption of new technologies in new areas, such as 'micro-electronics, bio-technology, advanced chemicals, new materials, computer applications, energy and communications systems', which required a 'highly skilled, better educated, and more mobile workforce' consisting of a 'large number of professional and technical staff' who would be supported by a 'range of highly trained workers performing a multitude of tasks rather than repetitive assembly or manufacture of a specific product'.

The target of this problematisation were young people between the ages of 11 and 18, and the aim was to keep them in full-time education beyond the age of 16. Full-time education was constructed as offering 'a better preparation for working life' through the availability of 'vocationally relevant courses'. The means by which this was to be achieved was through inclusion of a technical and vocational focus in the school curriculum in line with the emerging markets of the post-industrial society, the reconstitution of the role of the 'teacher' to fulfil the demands of the altered curriculum, reform of the examination system to allow for surveillance and measurement of the young person's 'achievements' and a system for surveillance and measurement of achievement of the aims of the altered curriculum.

Differing Dimensions of the Scottish Apparatus of Education

The particular technologies of this emerging discourse were divergent across English and Scottish contexts, reflecting the differing elements of the apparatus in which the discourse emerged. In a Scottish context, the discourse of vocational training emerged within a shifting policy agenda that allowed for the reconstitution of technologies of assessment to allow 'every pupil' to obtain recognition for his or her achievements (Scottish Education Department, 1988). The particular form the new technologies of assessment took were the 'standard grade' and the 'national certificate'. The 'standard grade' emerged against the problematisation of the 'O grade' as designed for 'high-achieving pupils' (Scottish Education Department, 1977), allowing for assessment of the new 'wider curriculum', one which would now have a focus on social and vocational skills, at three levels – foundation, general and credit – which aimed to cover the full range of pupils within the expanded school system. The 'national certificate' emerged against the problematisation of the 'bewildering choice' of qualifications and examining bodies faced by Scottish pupils (Scottish Education Department, 1983). In this new arrangement, learning could continue after leaving the school system, with 'modules' available through further education colleges, or the workplace, allowing for the national certificate to meet the needs of 'growing numbers of pupils for whom higher education was not an appropriate aim'.

This new arrangement of the apparatus of education can be argued to have the image of the active citizen of the post-industrial society as its aim. The new requirement for self-motivated self-enhancement in order to continually adapt to changing requirements of free market place is visible: the new requirement for 'life-long learning' was made possible through connecting schools, further education colleges and the workplace through the new modular system of examination. Additionally, the new forms of vocational training now available involved private enterprise in the delivery of the curriculum, allowing 'industry experts' to shape the curriculum in accordance with whatever demands the free market placed upon the worker. The new worker/citizen being fabricated would 'understand commercial culture [...] understand the profit motivation [...] understand about personal aspirations for personal success' (Kalms, 1988, cited in Gewirtz, Whitty, & Edwards, 1992) and would remedy the dependency culture of state welfare provision through doing things for themselves, thinking for themselves and acting responsibly.

Creating a New Background for the Active Young Person

A further element of the attempted enactment of the post-industrial society that offers clues to the shifting requirements of the citizen in this new configuration of society are 'enterprise zones'. The rationale for including these zones in this discussion are that they are considered to provide a glimpse of the background upon which the new active citizen would function and, thus, a glimpse of image that can be considered to be at the centre of the new requirements shaping the apparatus of education. The 'enterprise zone' first appeared within the Local Government Planning and Land Act (1980) and the Finance Act (1980). They can be considered as an 'experimental' enactment of New Right politico-economic rationalities which aimed to 'liberate enterprise throughout the country' through 'sensible deregulation' of the 'bureaucratic nightmare of rules and planning' that frustrates healthy private initiative.

Geographically, zones were designated areas that had experienced 'economic and physical decay' through the decline of earlier industrial or commercial activity, but rather than areas of high human cost, the zones targeted vacant land 'to test how far industrial and commercial activity could be encouraged by the removal or streamlining of administration of certain statutory or administrative controls'. Enterprise was to be attracted to the zones by a number of 'incentives', including a simplified planning regime, 100% allowance on corporation tax, exemption from development tax, exemption from paying rates on property, a reduction in official requests for governance information, exemption from contribution towards the costs of training workers and exemption from the requirement to supply information to industrial training boards.

Considered a 'New Right flagship', the enterprise zone can be considered as a microcosmic enactment of the post-industrial society, a glimpse of the materiality of the discourse. The 'incentives' were offered to attract business, with the aim being a property-led economic regeneration of the deindustrialised regions and the shifting of responsibility for their regeneration and the reversal of their economic and social problems from the state to the free market. The reduction in 'state controls' such as taxation and governance, and the proliferation of new 'arms-length' agencies and their involvement in administering the zones, can be considered to function as free market pockets, free from state involvement, where the 'invisible hand' of the free market would take over from the state in societal administration. To be a worker in these free market pockets required the ability to self-improve in line with the free market demands (there was no requirement for employers to train workers) and to be flexible to respond to the changing background; for those unwilling, or unable, there was no alternative (Thatcher, 1980); they would either self-improve or remain unemployed and governed by the new disciplining welfare apparatus.

Chapter 3: Part 2

The Material Effects of the 'Post-industrial Society': Inequality and Disadvantage

The promised shift from manufacturing to the third sector in the post-industrial society did not emerge in practice; between 1979 and 1983, in the UK, manufacturing output was reduced by approximately 28%, with the reduction in Scotland higher due to a higher concentration of heavy industry and manufacturing. In 1979, one-third of Scots worked in industry; by 1984, it was less than one-quarter. Scotland's manufacturing was reduced by approximately 30% with the three traditional mass employment sectors – shipbuilding, steel manufacturing and coal mining – all but wiped out. Over the same period, against losses of almost quarter of a million manufacturing jobs in Scotland, employment in the third sector increased by only 30,000. Additionally, the 'New Right flagship' enterprise zones, the 'experiment' in New Right societal administration, failed to create a free-market-driven economic recovery or produce employment for the 'active' citizen. Over a 10-year period, 38 zones were active, creating 126,000 jobs, with only 58,000 of these being classed as 'additional' jobs (see: Ward, 2016).

The differing employment figures illuminate an unintended effect of the zones: the relocation of enterprise from non-designated areas to the designated zones; and as the majority of the zones were designated in major cities, the result was concentrated job loss in smaller rural or semi-rural areas. An effect of this movement was that, whilst some previously industrial areas were reconfigured in line with the post-industrial discourse, most deindustrialised regions and the individuals who lived there were 'left to rot' (Anderson, 1990). The region in which this investigation was conducted can be considered as falling into this 'left to rot' category; it was not a designated enterprise zone, but it was geographically located near three of the four designated Scottish zones, and the material effects of the deindustrialisation are very clearly documented by the Office of National Statistics (2011) and the Scottish Public Health Observatory (2008) reports highlighted earlier. As I also outlined, the material effects also figured heavily in the conversations I had with the various local educational professionals; for example:

Excerpt 1:

> ***Family Support Worker:*** *I kind of... it scares me because... you know... having kind of gone out to work... well, left school in the Thatcher years... without kind of going and*

getting too political about it... and knowing what was available then. Which was nothing.

[...]

And it kind of feels like it's another cycle that we're going through, and when I first started working here it was great. There was money flying in... you know... because it's classed as an area of depravation... you know... there's drug use and... I mean, it's kind of inner city in a very rural area.

Excerpt 2:

Educational Psychologist: *I think in [region]... I think it was particularly hit because lots of industries would have closed all at once. It's a wee bit interesting community... and I call it a wee community on purpose I'm using those words fairly advisedly... it's a place where everybody knows everybody else and they're mostly related to each other as well. There are three distinct communities and they are notoriously suspicious of each other as well.*

[...]

The [area] cluster... and that's the cluster that I mostly cover... is very interesting because they're quite tight as a community. They've got lots of problems – massive social deprivation down there, huge social deprivation... but they're not the kind of folk... you know... you've got some other places where folk will say 'I haven't got' and 'I deserve' and 'it's my right'... the folk in [area] are not like that.

[...]

So I know, for example, in one of the primary schools where they would have a very high free school meal school meal entitlement, quite a lot of the parents don't claim it. They don't want help from outsiders. They don't want that kind of dependence. It's very... it's very odd actually. You would think that... you know... there's huge poverty and deprivation... you'd think you'd be saying 'yes please'. But no, they're quite close.

Excerpt 3:

Teacher 1: *I think it's about parenting. I think it's about attachment. I think it's about trauma. I think it's about... like*

I say... domestic abuse, substance abuse... you know... I think there's drugs and alcohol within [region]... you know the things that are known to have that...

Teacher 2: *You look at the health profiles it's poor. It's really quite shocking... you know... what the prospects are for our children, certainly for some of them... it's quite alarming.*

Interviewer: *It's quite a high area of deprivation, isn't it?*

Teacher 1: *We've got about 40% on decile one and two [lowest two indicators of family income].*

Within our school, yeah.

Interviewer: *In this school?*

Teacher 1: *In this school. So that's about two hundred kids to us... that's a big number in a school of five hundred.*

Interviewer: *So it's almost half of your cohort then?*

Teacher 1: *Yes, living in that... that level... in poverty and deprivation.*

Excerpt 4:

Deputy Head Teacher: *It's, umm... I mean, it's pretty grim. I would say their perception of it is there's... I mean traditionally... you know... the industries that were here... you know... the brewery and all that have gone. There is a high level of unemployment in [area], particularly [area], and the bottom end and out in [area]. Also because it's the smallest authority there is not the same... you know... facilities here for young people. But I think there is a push... you know... they're trying to develop a skate park now... there's different things... there is some kind of regeneration of the communities going on. But I do think that... you know... young people here feel that it's dead easy just to avoid it. They can... you know... take drugs, get wasted with your pals... you know... there's not an awful lot to do here. There's still quite a high level of unemployment... you know... in comparison... but they would probably answer that better than I would. But I think young people feel they do... they all say... you know... it's not [city], it's not is not [city], we don't have access to the same opportunities as other young people do.*

Educated and Unemployed: Increasing the Requirement for Education without Jobs

Along with the increasing deprivation outlined above, several effects specific to young people were also conditioned by the attempted enactment of the post-industrial society. The twin elements of the changing curriculum and welfare entitlement removal for young people resulted in increased numbers in the school system who would have previously left school at 16, and for whom further education was not a priority. It was difficult to find official statistics on this issue – I contacted the Scottish government requesting sources of data but was informed that statistics were not available for this time period; however, one study investigating the impact of the education reforms (Sinclair, Ironside, & Seifert, 1996) found that secondary school class sizes increased by 7.5%, pupil-teacher ratios reducing by 6.4% and class sizes of over 30 increasing by 5.4% nationally. In a Scottish context, the increase in secondary school pupil numbers was considerably larger, with an increase 18% occurring between 1983 and 1994 (Paterson, 1997).

Despite the increasing school pupil numbers and educational focus on vocational training, the destination for these young people was not employment in the new technology driven free market as intended. By 1989, approximately half the young people who engaged in vocational training were on government administered Youth Training Schemes, 30% were unemployed, with 20% in full-time employment outside schemes administered through governmental unemployment services (see: Bell, Howieson, King, & Raffe, 1989). At the same time, engagement in vocational training did not impact on employability, with the presence of vocational training experience not having a corresponding influence on the practices of recruitment and selection of enterprise; statements from employers can be seen to indicate that experience of vocational training would not influence selection of new employees. The effect of this shift towards vocational training, rather than the creation of a highly trained, vocationally able young workforce, was the maintenance of young people within the apparatus of education for longer and the creation of a subgroup of skilled young people, without employment opportunity, administered through governmental unemployment services, such as Youth Training Schemes or unemployment services, alongside the large numbers of adults classed as long-term unemployed.

Social Exclusion and Marginalisation of Young People

A further effect from the deindustrialisation was the exponential increase in young people socially excluded from society. The removal of welfare entitlements for young people under the age of 18, and restriction of entitlements for young people under the age of 25, resulted in large numbers of young people, unwilling to be governed by the discourses of vocational training, being marginalised from society. In *Learning to Labour*, Willis (1977) explores how the young people of the study 'get working class jobs' (p. 1) by documenting the discourses and practices that shaped the subjectivities required for taking up employment in the manufacturing industries. A dominant discourse in this process was that education was pointless and only for middle-class kids. The effect of the discourse was the devaluing of educational effort resulting in academic underachievement and leaving school at 16 for employment in manufacturing. The same discourse was apparent in this project, appearing in an account of the impact of deindustrialisation on the region by the same educational professional who highlighted the region's past prosperity. In the account, she recalls her own experience of schooling and educational choices:

> *I mean I had people in my family when I said that I wanted to go to university; they were kind of looking at me saying why do you want to do that? You know what you're going to do as a woman – sorry dad [whispering that to him up there] – was well you'll go and you'll do secretarial training and then you'll go and get an admin job and – you know – that's what you'll do, because then you'll get married and you'll have babies and you'll give up your work and – you know. So what was the point of – you know – going to university? My cousin's friends who did that because that – that's exactly what they did because there was still loads of these industries around that required the typing pool and the admin skills and things like that. So the desire for further education and higher education wasn't huge because there were plenty of job opportunities for sensible, competent people to do straight after school.*
>
> *[...].*
>
> *So my generation kind of had to think differently about what they were going to do at the end of education but maybe people just five years before me, they could do a reasonable spread 1st to 4th year, keep your nose clean, don't get into too much trouble, and then leave school and get a job.*

In the midst of the deindustrialisation of the local area, this would have not have resulted in employment in working-class jobs, or even in unemployment, but in the creation of subgroups of young people not in receipt of welfare assistance and not appearing in official unemployment statistics. As these young people were excluded from official statistics, it is impossible to gauge the numbers of young people marginalised by this process; however, if one considers the emergence of the category of NEET in the construction of this particular group of young people as a social problem, as several critics have argued (see: Bynner & Parsons, 2002; Crisp & Powell, 2017; Furlong, 2006; Melrose, 2012), then an indication of the 'scale of the problem of NEET' suggests that, by the early 1990s, approximately 9% (161,000) of 16- to 17-year-olds per year were being socially excluded from society (see: Social Exclusion Unit, 1999b).

Invariably, though, dominant contemporary discourses of youth unemployment do not construct NEET as the result of punitive welfare reforms aimed at 'encouraging' continued education or take-up of vocational training, but as the result of lacking the personal characteristics deemed necessary to fulfil the societal obligation of work, reflecting the transmutation of social issues into moral problems by New Right politico-economic discourse.

Chapter 4: Part 1

Governing Young People through 'Additional Support for Learning'

In the previous chapter, I provided an overview of the changing politico-economic background of the region and the changing requirements of the young person that emerged from within this process. The chapter was made possible by the discussions that informed this chapter and, thus, these are important for foregrounding this chapter. As stated at the start of the previous chapter, this shifting background is important because of what was made possible in the present. The effects created – particularly poverty and disadvantage and the emerging role of the apparatus of education in shaping the future citizen – are considered important in conditioning the elements expanded upon in this chapter: 'social inclusion' as requirement of schools and the emergence of 'additional support needs' as a category of disability.

Both of these elements are considered an important focus in this investigation as their intersecting genealogical lines can be seen to have created the conditions for the invention of a grid of procedures, knowledges and technologies for 'supporting' young people 'to' learn. My argument is that this grid emerged as a solution to a proliferation of 'learning problems' conditioned by the emergence of social inclusion as a strategic aim of the apparatus of education and a requirement to meet the learning needs of every pupil required by policies regarding additional support needs. It is the appearance of this grid, conditioned by these intersecting elements, that is considered to have allowed for an increase in use of psychiatric knowledge within the school.

This chapter, like the last, is offered in two sections. In the first section, I chart two genealogical lines – one for social inclusion and one for additional support needs – tracking backwards from their appearance within the apparatus of education. In the first genealogical line, I chart the appearance of social inclusion as a strategic aim of the education of apparatus through Scottish and UK political discourse, connecting this with the emergence of 'Third-Way' politics. In the second genealogical line, I chart the expansion of the category of disability, illuminating the changing requirements conditioned by its reconstitution from a discrete biological condition to 'anything' that has a bearing on educational progress. In the second section of the chapter, I provide an analysis of the emergence of ADHD as an explanation within the grid of procedures, knowledges and technologies conditioned by the intersecting elements charted in part 1 of the chapter.

Genealogical Line 1: Social Exclusion as Problematisation of the 'Effects' of Deindustrialisation

The appearance of social exclusion/inclusion as a problem and focus of political discourse in the UK can be connected to emergence of 'Third Way' politics, with its stated aims of combining social solidarity with a dynamic economy. The problem of social exclusion has a longer history, however, originating in French political discourse in the 1960s and 1970s. Within this discursive framework, social exclusion has as its target citizens separated from mainstream society by disability, illness and poverty, with social and economic rather than individual factors constructed as the cause of exclusion. Considered to be informed by French republicanism, the concern for the socially excluded connects to the concepts of solidarity, the social bond and equity for all citizens that structured French societal organisation.

In UK political discourse, however, the problem of social exclusion lacks a clear target, with concepts such as 'multiple deprivation' and 'complex inequality' presented as its concern. This vagueness is visible in various statements constructing descriptions of the unit tasked with tackling social exclusion that is considered the beginning of its emergence as a problem within UK political discourse. The social exclusion unit (SEU), a 'flagship' policy invention attributable to 'Third Way' political discourse, constructs social exclusion as occurring because of 'prospects and networks and life chances': as a 'modern problem', as 'damaging to the self-esteem of the individual' and as 'what can happen when people or areas suffer from a combination of linked problems such as unemployment, poor skills, low incomes, poor housing, high crime, poor health and family breakdown' (see: Blair, 1997; Social Exclusion Unit, 2004a). The discourse of the SEU also positions social exclusion as resulting from 'wider demographic and economic changes', particularly those from the '1980s and 1990s', and caused by 'poverty and low income; unemployment; poor school results; poor mental or physical health; family breakdown and poor parenting; poor housing and homelessness; discrimination; crime; and living in a disadvantaged area' (Social Exclusion Unit, 2004b, p. 13).

The characteristics of the SEU social exclusion discourse – particularly the focus on the wider demographic and economic factors of the 1980s and 90s as involved in poverty, unemployment, poor school results, poor mental or physical health, poor housing, etc. – imply a UK version of a French republican discourse, one that conveys concern for solidarity and the social bond and equality for all citizens. However, the target of UK political discourse, despite the connection to wider demographic and economic factors, was on social groups and *their* problems, rather than on the political and economic background. This is clearly emphasised in the constructed solutions: social exclusion would be tackled through provision of equal opportunity for all and elimination of barriers to these opportunities, which would be achieved through the provision of the individual skills and attributes required to reconnect the *individual* with the labour market. This focus is also visible in various statements presented by the SEU: 'the best defence against social exclusion is having a job, and the best way to get a job is to have a good education, with the right training and experience' (Social Exclusion Unit, 1999a, p. 6). In this construction, the individual and their skills, abilities and attributes remain the problem and cause of social exclusion and, thus, the focus of intervention. However, rather than being because of a moral and behavioural deficiency, as was dominant in UK political discourse in the 1980s, the lack of attributes was positioned as resulting from missing out on opportunity due to social exclusion.

Scottish Devolution and the Emergence of Social 'Inclusion'

A variation of social exclusion can be seen in flagship policies of the first devolved Scottish government. In a raft of policies targeting the 'problems' of Scottish society, social *inclusion* is positioned as the opposite of social exclusion, as the means of tackling exclusion and as the central aim of post-devolved Scottish political policy. Social exclusion remains a multi-dimensional problem: as caused by a 'broad range of social problems, centred around low income, lack of opportunity, diminished quality of life and degraded environments' and as 'what can happen when individuals or areas suffer from a combination of linked problems such as unemployment, poor skills, low incomes, poor housing, high crime environments, bad health and family breakdown' (p. 8). To solve the problem, a new configuration of institutions and professionals would promote social inclusion through participation in the labour market, which would be achieved by tackling the specific barriers to participation that *individuals* faced, including 'ill health, low self-esteem, homelessness and drug misuse' and by promoting 'a culture of active citizenship, in which self-development, participation in community and civic life and caring for our disadvantaged neighbours' (p. 8) were key features.

Within UK political discourse, exclusion and inclusion can be considered to have shifted from their French republican origins: the problematisation of exclusion as resulting from social and economic factors gives way to a problematisation of individual attributes (Levitas, 2005; Silver, 2010). In this new focus, individuals are positioned as socially excluded because they lack the education, training or skills required for employment. There is also a silencing of the wider political and economic background implicated in social exclusion: the individual barriers that result in social exclusion are constructed as *because of social exclusion*, with education, training and employment constructed as the pathway out of disadvantage and towards *social inclusion*. This particular shift can be seen as decontextualising and depoliticising the material effects of political and economic approach of 1980s and 1990s allowing for a continued targeting of the individual as the solution. However, in this approach, the deployment of disciplining measures, such as stripping of welfare rights and creation of mass unemployment, can be seen to give way to an approach to governance that requires active engagement from individuals. In this new approach, individual active involvement is encouraged, not through punishment and coercion, but through a pastoral approach, one that positions social exclusion as holding the individual back from doing well in life where, if they are able and willing to engage with state-provided opportunities to self-improve, the result will be social *inclusion* and a pathway out of disadvantage. In this new construction, individuals who continued to be socially *excluded* remain so, not because of political and economic structures, but because they, as individuals, have not taken advantage of the opportunities made available to them to 'take part in work, in learning, and in society more generally' (Scottish Office Education and Industry Department, 1999).

Shaping the Young Person through Inclusion: The Case of Education

The particular construction of social inclusion outlined above – one that depoliticises exclusion, positions it as the cause of disadvantage, and constructs individual engagement with state-provided opportunities as the pathway to inclusion – also emerges within the apparatus of education, highlighting the positioning of education as a technology for its enactment. In the document outlined earlier – 'Social Inclusion: Opening the Door to a Better Scotland' – education is positioned as the 'best way to achieve a significant, long-term difference to the incidence of social exclusion' (Scottish Office Education and Industry Department, 1999, p. 6), as this would 'develop [the young person's] skills and their employability' (Scottish Office Education and Industry Department, 1999, p. 5) with the individual young person positioned as having 'responsibility for making the most of those opportunities' (Scottish Office Education and Industry Department, 1999, p. 5). These particular aims – the construction of a skilled, employable and responsibilised young person – can be seen as a continuation of the activisation of the young citizen through the apparatus of education outlined in the previous chapter. However, the incorporation of the discourse of social inclusion can be considered to allow for the shift in the functioning of power, from one that excluded 'problems' to one that would function through technologies of inclusion and normalisation.

This changing educational background was illuminated in an interview with a deputy head teacher. In the following excerpt, he provides a description of a separate school domain where young people were sent once categorised as problematic by mainstream school. The role of the domain appears to function solely as a space to banish 'problems' from mainstream school, possibly acting as an intermediary step to more coercive forms of exclusion (residential school). In this domain, education and learning was not a central concern of the exclusion process, with teaching and learning missing from the account of the activities. In the second part of the account, excerpt 2, the deputy head documents the shift to inclusion and the proliferation of technologies, and associated professionals, that functioned as part of a network for including young people, considered problematic, within mainstream schools. This new focus and approach can be seen to have emerged within the shifting requirements of the apparatus of education which now aimed to 'support' young people in their learning within the mainstream school.

Excerpt 1:

> ***Interviewer:*** *I presume that's what you were saying about just coming down and there wasn't the education side of things –*
> ***Deputy head teacher:*** *Aye. I think it's started off – you come down – you know – play a couple of songs, play pool, they used to smoke and all that... you know... way back in 1970 when it was set up and it was just a resources thing for keeping kids out of residential school at that point... because it was a different way of thinking.*

Excerpt 2:

> ***Deputy head teacher:*** *Within each of the three mainstream schools they have a behaviour support department who are primarily staffed by a senior member of staff and learning assistants who will...*
>
> ***Interviewer:*** *So they're teachers the... the heads of these places?*
>
> ***Deputy head teacher:*** *Yeah. They would be teachers. But the people who run it tend to be... sorry the people who support it, would tend to be kind of learning assistants. They run very differently in each of the three secondary schools.*
>
> *[...]*
>
> *So there are behavioural supports they all have a range of strategies that they'll try and employ within schools through behaviour cards or active timetables to support a young person. But – and then you've also got the learning support department or the additional support needs department which is more about young people's learning. So young people come down there and they would get a hand with their schoolwork but they're very different in each of the three schools.*

Genealogical Line 2: Thinning the Mesh and Widening the Net: The Changing Category of Disability

The current category of disability functioning within the apparatus of education – additional support needs – is a relatively new category of school-based disability, with its appearance and functioning within the apparatus traceable to the Education (Additional Support for Learning) (Scotland) Act (2004). This new category positioned additional support needs as anything that acted as a 'barrier to learning' and placed the requirement for meeting the needs with mainstream schools. This is considered an important shift in the discursive background of the apparatus of education, one that can be considered to intersect with and be legitimated by the appearance of social inclusion as a strategic aim of education. However, the appearance of disability in this particular form at this historical juncture warrants consideration as its gradual transformation across several policies can be seen to have conditioned the possibility for the intersection with the social inclusion agenda charted above. The starting point for this account is the 'Special Education Needs: Report of the Committee of Enquiry into the Education of Handicapped Children and Young People, The Warnock Report'. The Warnock Report is considered an important element in this changing background as its recommendations were codified in the Education Scotland Act (1981), which in turn conditioned the possibility for the current procedures for managing 'problems' in Scottish schools to be codified as additional support needs.

Prior to the enactment of the Warnock Report, biological and medical discourse provided the procedures for the management of 'problems' within the apparatus of education, visible in the various subcategories that constituted the Education (Scotland) Act (1945) classification of 'handicapped'. Each of the 11 subcategories – blind, partially sighted, deaf, partially deaf, delicate, diabetic, educationally subnormal, epileptic, maladjusted, physically handicapped, and speech defects – constructed problems as an innate disability, biological in origin and as requiring certification through 'medical examination' by a 'medical officer' in order to receive either specialist education 'treatment' or certification as 'suffering from a disability of mind or body' (Warnock, 1978, p. 28) and as incapable of receiving education. The category of 'handicapped', and the requirement for education authorities to provide specialist educational 'treatment' for this new category, legitimated a proliferation of specialist educational settings, the classification of large numbers of young people as 'handicapped' and for exclusion to function as a means for managing 'problems' of learning.

The problematisation of segregated specialist education is apparent in the changing category for classification of disability that appears in the Warnock Report. In the report, the category of 'handicapped' is reconstituted as 'special education needs', vaguely defined as an incapacity or disadvantage that hindered learning, as on a continuum and as ranging in form and severity. The shift from 'handicapped' to 'special education needs' is legitimated through deployment of 'evidence' from newly emergent child and adolescent epidemiological studies.[1] The 'problem' considered by these studies was young people considered not to be doing well educationally despite not being considered to be 'handicapped' (i.e. those in mainstream school performing badly). The reality constructed was

[1]See: Rutter, Tizard, Yule, Graham, and Whitmore (Isle of Wight Studies, 1976).

that there was no distinction between 'handicapped' and other concepts, such as 'disability', 'incapacity' and 'disadvantage', and that the relationship between handicap in educational terms and the severity of a disability in social terms was more complex than initially thought. In this new reality of disability, the school environment was positioned as key to whether disabilities would contribute to poor educational outcomes: if school adjusted to the disability, the young person would not be educationally 'handicapped'.

This new reality of disability can be seen to have legitimated a widening of what could be constituted as disability, allowing for a shift from targeting discrete 'biological defects' to any form of incapacity or disadvantage that could hinder educational outcomes. This new consideration of what constituted disability expanded the category from its confinement by biological discourse to include social, emotional and behavioural dimensions. A material effect of this shift was an increase in what could be constructed as 'special needs'. Special educational needs were now considered to relate to 'everything about [the young person], his abilities as well as his disabilities – indeed all the factors which have a bearing on his educational progress' (Warnock, 1978, p. 37), allowing for a shift from a system of discrete and permanent labels to one of fluidity and change: a dynamic system of educational surveillance and 'treatment'. This 'thinning of the mesh and widening of the net' (Cohen, 1979) can be considered to have increased the range of who could be targeted for intervention; the net was now wide enough to include any young person considered at risk of poor educational outcomes, with anything impacting on learning now considered legitimate for intervention.

A New Technology of Disability: Mainstream School

This shifting understanding of disability legitimated new procedures for the management of what was constructed as special needs. Previously, the categories of 'handicapped', once certified as such by medical examination, were fixed upon the young person by a medical authority, remaining fixed for the entirety of their time in the educational apparatus and beyond. Specialist education was prescribed as 'treatment', which took the form of segregation from mainstream schools in separate educational facilities specific to the form of disability assigned to the young person. However, with the emergence of the new fluid concept of special needs, the mainstream school was reconstituted as the means of management of this new category of disability. This new approach would require the mainstream school to adjust educational provision to meet the specific learning problems of young people, and would extend to locational, social, functional and academic domains of the school experience.

The shift from exclusion and specialist schooling to inclusion and mainstream schooling was legitimated by this new form of disability. As discussed above, the Warnock R problematises the category of 'handicapped' as not being wide enough to capture the full extent of the problems of learning that were considered to be present in the school population. Through application of the wider concept of special education needs, the Warnock Report calls for special education needs to be expanded to one in five of the school population (Warnock, 1978, p. 41). These needs were to be considered as time-limited problems of learning, as stemming from a 'variety of causes' rather than 'handicapped in the traditional sense of the term' and, without time-limited suitable help, the problems would be 'reinforced by prolonged experience of failure' (Warnock, 1978, p. 41).

By expanding the category to cover young people not considered to be handicapped but not doing well in *mainstream* school, the new construction problematises mainstream school educational provision as not being adequate enough to meet 'less noticeable forms of disability' experienced by one of five of the pupil population. The beginnings of a preventative discourse can also be detected in this new construction – these needs would be 'time limited' if provision was made to remedy the variety of causes from which they stemmed, which included the contribution of the school environment to the problems. The implicit construction is that these less noticeable disabilities would be avoided if schools adapted provision early in order to reduce the 'prolonged' failure experienced by this previously silent group of young people.

This new reality of educational disability and its inclusion in mainstream school constructed in and legitimated by the Warnock Report became codified by the Education Act (1981) in England and Wales and the Education (Scotland) Act (1981), further legitimating by law the expanded category of special education needs. Both acts codified the requirement for education authorities to assess the educational needs of young people considered to have difficulties with learning and for these to be recorded and monitored as a 'Statement' in England and Wales and a 'Record of Needs' in Scotland. A key divergence between these two acts, however, was that the English and Welsh act codified the requirement for inclusion in mainstream schools, whereas the Scottish legislation did not make such a commitment. Both sets of legislation construct special education needs in line with the wider focus legitimised by the Warnock Report and codify the requirement for special education *provision*; however, the English legislation placed a requirement for the provision to be made in ordinary school (Education Act, 1981, p. 2), whereas the Scottish legislation restricted the requirement to the expedient identification of young people with special educational needs, provision of suitable forms of education for meeting these needs and continued surveillance of both needs and provision thereafter (Education (Scotland) Act, 1981, pp. 12–15). As such, within the Scottish educational apparatus, exclusion remained a technology for managing problems of learning, with the reach of its application expanded to meet the wider category of special education needs; however, its continued functioning was time limited, eventually problematised by the Standards in Scotland's Schools etc. Act (2000) as a contributing factor to the social exclusion and disadvantage visible in Scottish society.

The solution proposed by the Standards in Scotland's Schools etc. Act was the placement of a 'requirement for mainstreaming education' for every pupil, placing responsibility for education of young people considered to have special educational needs on mainstream schools, with education to be adapted to meet their specific abilities. The new requirement of mainstream education for all pupils irrespective of disability was legitimated by a moralising discourse, one that positioned social exclusion and disadvantage as an individual problem that resulted from poor education and urged those providing education to be more adaptive in order to contribute to solving the problem. The requirement for mainstream education was connected to social exclusion by reconstituting disability as relating to differing 'personal or social circumstances' that acted as obstacles to education and, thus, to future well-being. Removing these obstacles was now a 'duty' as it would provide 'equity' in education provision and, thus, equity of opportunity for everyone regardless of circumstances. By including everyone regardless of difference, the 'belief they mattered' would 'instilled' in the young person, encouraging them towards achieving the highest possibilities available to them based on *individual* abilities and strengths. This requirement to 'achieve' was presented as beneficial not only to those considered to have special education needs but to all pupils, the whole school and society generally, as educated and achieving young people would provide a 'significant contribution to the economic growth of the country, improving well-being, family life, lifestyles, communities and the nation as a whole' (Scottish Government, 2017, pp. 16–17). This new reality of an adaptive education system that met the needs of everyone positioned inclusion as beneficial to everyone; this contrasts with the reality of exclusion authorised by the Education (Scotland) Act (1945), where exclusion of those constructed as 'handicapped' from the mainstream school was considered beneficial to those who remained in the mainstream school.

Expanding the Continuum of Need: The Inclusion of Complex Needs

The category of 'special education needs' was reconstituted as 'additional support' needs by the Education (Additional Support for Learning) (Scotland) Act (2004). In terms of what it could target, the new category was similar in focus to the category it replaced, with both constructed as the solution to the problem of obstacles that impacted on learning and achievement. Similar to special education needs, the new category, by providing equity in educational provision through recognising 'individuals' challenges and barriers to learning', and by putting in place additional provision, would ensure that young people considered to have additional support needs would be 'given the best possible chance of being a full part of society' (Scottish Parliament Education Committee, 2003; col. 564). This new category also allowed for a variety of school-based problems to be constructed as additional support needs if, 'for whatever reason', the young person is, 'or is likely to be', unable without the provision of additional support, to benefit from school education (Education (Additional Support for Learning) (Scotland) Act 2004, p. 1).

Where additional support needs differed, however, was the inclusion of 'complex needs' within its reach. As outlined above, the category of special education needs was legitimated on claims of the existence of problems of learning that were too subtle to be 'picked up' by the previous procedures legitimated by the category of 'handicapped'. The reality created was that there were less noticeable forms of disability that were not being 'treated' and that mainstream school was not meeting the needs of this hidden population and was thus contributing to the poor educational outcomes of this group of young people. The new category of additional support needs, however, now required mainstream schools to meet needs arising from 'one or more *complex* factors' or 'multiple factors' (Additional Support for Learning) (Scotland) Act 2004, p. 2), with 'factors' vaguely defined as anything 'likely to have a significant adverse effect on the school education' (Additional Support for Learning) (Scotland) Act 2004, p. 2).

The inclusion of complexity in this new category legitimated a shift in the means by which barriers to learning would be reduced. The category of special education needs would support learning through 'adjustments in current mainstream provision', with the adjustments – and thus the problems of learning – considered as 'time limited'. However, the new category of additional support needs expanded what would be required to be provided by mainstream schools, from time limited adjustments for low-level special education needs to 'significant additional support', which would be required to 'continue for more than a year' (Additional Support for Learning) (Scotland) Act 2004, p. 2). To meet this expanded requirement within its remit, mainstream schools would now require involvement of 'one or more appropriate agencies', with 'appropriate agencies' defined as local authority and health board departments. Inclusion of the wider network in meeting problems of learning would be authorised by the school – involvement would be defined as appropriate if it could 'help in the exercise of any of the education authority's functions', with individual schools required to specify what was required to meet additional support needs (Additional Support for Learning) (Scotland) Act 2004, p. 18).

Chapter 4: Part 2

The 'Official' Procedures of Inclusion and Additional Support Needs

The genealogical accounts in the first part of this chapter are important for discursively positioning the emergence of the current procedures for managing problems of learning in the schools that were described in the interviews with educational professionals. The question that informed the interviews asked about how schools responded to learning problems and how ADHD was recognised and processed from within these procedures. I was interested in what was *done* – i.e. the knowledges, techniques and procedures deployed in the management of school-based problems – in order to understand how these came to be in place and how they contributed to young people being constructed as 'having' ADHD.

Through these conversations, an extensive grid of procedures, knowledges and technologies for making problems of learning intelligible was made visible, one that expanded across nursery education, primary schools, secondary schools and outwards to health and social service agencies. The 'official' representation of the grid was laid out in material that was provided to parents and young people, with a similar account offered in an interview with an educational professional. Both are positioned below for comparison:

Official Procedure	Professional Account
Stage 1 Teachers and nursery staff may recognise that the child or young person may need some short-term changes or support to help them get the best out of the work in the group or class. The supports will be reviewed and the child can be removed from Stage 1 or moved to Stage 2 if further help is needed. Parents/carers are informed and kept actively involved.	***Educational psychologist:*** *So Stage 1 is a kind of monitoring stage where things are starting to bubble away, school are just like, right, OK, but there's no external agency involved and it's really just right, OK, we need to make some tweaks in-house.* *Stage 2 is a sort of assessment stage, where things are starting to increase a little bit and they're starting to think about we might want to bring in the primary school support service outreach, we might want to bring in inclusion therapists, we might want to start*

(*Continued*)

Official Procedure	**Professional Account**
Stage 2 A meeting will be held with the parents/carers and where possible, the child or young person. Other staff may also be invited, i.e. family support workers, support for learning staff etc. A plan will be put in place to address the child or young person's additional support needs. The plan is agreed and reviewed at least annually. Following a Stage 2 review the child or young person may continue on Stage 2, return to Stage 1 or move to Stage 3 if more support is needed. **Stage 3** A planned move to Stage 3 will happen due to a need to individualise aspects of the child or young person's curriculum. One or more specialists or agencies could be involved, i.e. speech and language therapist, social workers, outreach staff, educational psychologists, offering support in a more direct role. An Individualised Educational Programme (IEP) will be drawn up with short- and long-term targets to be achieved by the child or young person. The IEP targets will be reviewed; short-term targets are normally reviewed every term and long-term targets every year. At the annual Stage 3 review the child or young person may remain at Stage 3 with new targets developed, or they may return to Stage 2, or a request can be made to the Staged Intervention Scrutiny Group for a move to Stage 4.	*having – you know – raising this name with the educational psychologist.* *[...]* **Interviewer:** Who does the assessment? ***Educational psychologist:*** *It's done within the schools.* **Interviewer:** So, like a teacher-led thing? ***Educational psychologist***: *Yeah, yeah. So when we've got – at the point where we become involved – we usually become involved through a team around the child meeting. School might say wee Jimmy is having difficulty with X, Y, or Z – are you available to come along to a consultation?* *[...]* *So, now with the consultation model, you either open it and close it straight away, or you open it because you're going to do a specific piece of assessment or intervention. So we tend to go along to the team around the child meeting, we have a consultation document that we complete that has various different bits of information on it – it's quite functional: name, address, date of birth – and what we think the concerns are. And then on the back page we have an action plan we share with whoever's been involved in the consultation. So consultation can take place just with the class teacher, or the head or the depute, or it could be a full team around the child meeting.* *[...]* *So at that point we make a decision as to whether or not we just are involved on a consultation basis as a one-off, so – you know – you might provide some*

(*Continued*)

Official Procedure	Professional Account
Stage 4 Following agreement by the Staged Intervention Scrutiny Group a child or young person will be moved to Stage 4 where there is need for an extensive degree of individualisation, adaptation or enhancement of the curriculum and/or learning environment. There will also be a number of specialists and/or agencies involved. An IEP will be in place and in some cases, a coordinated support plan (CSP). Parents/carers and the child or young person will be involved in meetings and decision making. A Stage 4 review will take place at least once a year.	*psycho-education around whatever – you know – you might have resources that you hand out – it's an open/closed case.* *[...]* *Within schools – within the staged intervention process, we have a set of paperwork that schools are expected to complete to track children. All children will have – they have different names – but things like a personal learning plan. And that's every school – that's the universal level – so every child will have something that says 'this is wee Jimmy and they're working on X, Y and Z – you know – this is how he did on it'. Children who become more involved in the staged intervention process will have what we call an individual education plan, where they have specific targets that they're working on.* *[...]* *So that's at the level of – you know – kids who are getting to the sort of stage three in staged intervention, they should have a child's plan.* *[...]* *But then you get another layer above it which is the coordinated support plan. And coordinated support plan is a legal document and there's specific assessment periods and paperwork that goes with it. There's specific criteria for children to meet to say that they need a coordinated support plan, which is generally that it requires the coordination of agencies external to education. So things like health services, social work, voluntary agencies – that they need to be coordinated in such a way to meet the educational needs of the child.*

(*Continued*)

Official Procedure	Professional Account
	So, for example, the cases where we most often have CSPs would be the children who attend things like extended ESN – persevere in complex provision – so for them to be able to meet their educational goals, they need support from, for example, the physiotherapist to provide them with equipment to be able to get into school and things like that. And those needs need to be substantial and last for longer than a year.

The existence and purpose of the grid was conditioned by the new requirement for mainstream schools to support *every* child and young person to learn irrespective of disability codified by the Education (Additional Support for Learning) (Scotland) Act (2004). The requirement for a 'staged/tiered' approach to management of school-based problems was outlined in official policy, but the specifics of the approach were to be developed by each region (Scottish Government, 2003, p. 91). Both 'official' and professional accounts of the grid enacted locally construct the image of an approach that adapts the school environment, including the curriculum, to the young person's specific needs, with these adaptations based on careful assessment of risk to learning. The inclusion discourse is visible in both accounts: depending on assessment, the problem would be placed on the grid, with 'tweaks in house' at the lowest level to an 'extensive degree of individualisation, adaptation or enhancement of the curriculum and/or learning environment' at the highest level, being made to adjust the school environment to individual needs, allowing the grid to include and manage the full continuum of needs within its reach.

A preventative discourse is also present in the accounts. The requirement for adaptations to be reviewed on a regular basis, with movement back down (or up if required) the continuum of need if the problem had reduced through the support offered, indicates that problems are not considered fixed but could be remedied through the grid of intervention. The forms of knowledge for understanding school-based problems that permeated the grid are positioned as holistic, with dominant explanations structured by discourses of attachment or trauma; in these explanations, developmental history and context are considered important for understanding the problem:

Excerpt 1:

> **Teacher:** *We're dealing with the child in front of us, so therefore it's the behaviours that we see on a day-to-day – and obviously dependent on the relationship with the class*

teacher – you know – often the dynamics of the class – there's so many different factors that can determine how a child's managing within the school environment.

Interviewer: *So you wouldn't immediately assume ADHD then –*

Teacher: *No. Not at all. I would say especially not –*

Teacher 2: *...I would say especially not.*

Teacher: *No, I think a lot of – we look at attachment – probably... for us, that would be one of the things that often comes up –*

Excerpt 2:

Interviewer: *So who takes them on depends on the type of assessment that occurs? I suppose that then would influence what happens next.*

Educational psychologist: *In some ways, yeah. I think – you know – we've been having discussions sort of informally – we haven't got to the level of having a sort of formal team meeting, but the landscape's changing. You know, there's going to be less of us going forward because they're not going to turn into an increase in our numbers – I would be very surprised if that was the case. We're obviously now splitting from [region] and things like that. And we've had sort of initial discussions just amongst ourselves but to say actually do we need to split ourselves and say right, we've got a learning team, and we've got an attachments team, for example – or attachment and trauma because a lot of us are trained in more specific attachment –*

Excerpt 3:

Educational psychologist: *So for a while we had [name] heading up the intervention project from Western European Social Fund money, so he had [name] and then we had three Early Years workers.*

Interviewer: *Right.*

Educational psychologist: *And the Early Years workers part of that disappeared, and we just had [name] providing a therapeutic input.*

Interviewer: *And that was attachment work – from an attachment perspective – or – ?*

Educational psychologist: *Attachment and trauma. So he would use – you know – Dan Hughes Dyadic Developmental Psychotherapy – he would use that approach, but he would also do a lot of EMDR work with people who'd been traumatised, abused, whatever.*

In this holistic, supportive and inclusive system, the requirement for diagnosis generally, and ADHD specifically, was not considered to be required – needs would determine provision, rather than specific conditions or diagnoses. This was made clear by an educational psychologist I spoke with:

Interviewer: *Is there any benefit then to having the diagnosis of ADHD or ASD for the families?*

Educational psychologist: *From an education point of view, the answer should be no. And currently the answer is no. And I would hate to think that we would get to a point where it becomes a necessity. And in fact, actually a colleague and I were just talking about this before you came in, because under the Additional Support for Learning Act, we don't need a diagnosis. So, for example, this morning I was taking a family to visit the [school] ASD provision. Now their daughter is probably highly likely to get a diagnosis of ASD at some point, but she doesn't have one currently. But the process is set up in such a way that as long as the team around the child have a consensus, and actually we can see on paper the sort of things that she's having difficulty with, then we don't need a diagnosis. [...] And that's the same whether it's ASD, ADHD or whatever.*

This positioning of need over diagnosis was also presented in the accounts offered at the level of the school by teachers and a deputy head teacher (from different schools). Both professional groups were asked questions about how schools responded to learning problems and how ADHD was recognised and processed from within these problems. Both groups offered a similar response – that they did not see disorder when considering problems of learning:

Excerpt 1:

Interviewer: *I'm interested from a school's perspective. So, how would you recognise ADHD? You know, if you'd seen a child, how would you know that that was ADHD? Or what would make you think it was ADHD? And then what* *would you do about that? What are the processes that you would follow?*

Teacher: *I think first and foremost we don't make the judgment on whether we think a child has ADHD or not. What – I think we always look at children who perhaps present as very anxious or have a very poor attention span, or I don't know their ability – they seem very hyper and agitated. And we start to look at a bigger picture for that child, you know? So, for us the very initial steps we're gathering information around that, especially for a new child to the school, because we want to find out their background. We'd try to find out about home circumstances, whether there's been any involvement from any other agency prior – you now – previous to coming here, or whether they are still ongoing.*

Excerpt 2:

Interviewer: *Within the range of pupils you see in the kind of various ways in which they present – how would you interpret their behaviour?*

Deputy head: *I think we've kind of got – I mean I think – you know – we get young people with – or who have displayed quite extreme behaviour within a mainstream setting. Extreme behaviour for us in here would be kids picking up furniture and kind of launching it. And we don't see that often – that's kind of extreme.*

[…]

So we do a lot of work here building up relationships. A lot of our young people do get it wrong but they tend to get it wrong and it manifests itself and coming out as 'rarr rarr' – frustration, anger, and that's the kind of – that's your bread-and-butter – you know –

[…]

Interviewer: *So what do you think causes the behaviour – like, that type of behaviour?*

Deputy head: *I think in here a lot of the time it's frustration, it's trying to mask learning difficulties. I think some of the kids can just have a bad day before they've come to school.*

> *Sometimes it's about establishing themselves in the pecking order. Sometimes it's just playing up for their peers. So there's a whole range of kind of reasons and I think what we try and do is find out as quickly as we can – you know – what the reason is and try to help them solve it. Not necessarily finding out what the reason is – just helping the young person solve it and say, well, like you being a listener, they'll tell it to us – you can behave like this – so let's try and get there quickly – you know?*

However, despite what could be considered as resistance to ADHD, and diagnosing more generally, and a system that prioritises need over condition, where the environment would be adapted to meet the specific needs of a young person, there was recognition that ADHD diagnosis was increasing in prominence within the school system:

Excerpt 1:

> ***Teacher:*** *When you're seeing a child who for all of – you know – all of a sudden, it's presenting perhaps more anxious, more distressed, not coping within class, bit of challenge of behaviour, say – you might just think, I'm just going to call a meeting, because I just want all of us checking and hearing what's going on – has there been a sudden change – does someone know something we don't know. And that can be useful just to put like around a table.*
>
> ***Interviewer:*** *So that would be for any kind of issues, then? Not necessarily ADHD –*
>
> ***Teacher:*** *Mhmm. It could be.*
>
> ***Teacher 2:*** *It could be, yeah. That could be a wider issue. But again, if we were seeing a real decline in ability to attend to any task, for instance, that would be something we'd need to say, well, what's changed – why were they able to do that three weeks ago and then –*
>
> ***Teacher:*** *Again, my thinking would be that a child with ADHD would have always found that challenging – you know – would not suddenly become – so therefore on that occasion like you say you'd think something's changed – something else is going on – it's something else – whereas – you know – a child with those definite challenges – you'd expect to be seeing that –*

> ***Teacher 2:*** *I do feel that it's a diagnosis that's being made more often.*
>
> ***Interviewer:*** *Sorry?*
>
> ***Teacher 2:*** *I think it's a diagnosis that's being made more often. But for us it's maybe come as a surprise, because of – we might have said it would have perhaps been much more related to attachment, and – you know – and trauma.*

Excerpt 2:

> ***Interviewer:*** *So something like ADHD then, that type of behaviour that is considered that way – what sort of things would you do?*
>
> ***Educational psychologist:*** *At the assessment stage or the intervention stage?*
>
> ***Interviewer:*** *I suppose both, really. So the assessment would be get feedback from teachers, and then what?*
>
> ***EP:*** *Well, the assessment would be information from the school, gathering information from parents – you know – developmental – general developmental history is something that we – you know – really blindingly obvious or is there nothing. And covering things like divorce and separation. Trying to rule out is this an attachment difficulty. And then if you're coming down on the side of it being ADHD or a neuro-developmental difficulty, in terms of intervention, I don't know that we've got a – it's probably an area where we don't have a huge amount of resource. Because actually, until recently, ADHD wasn't something that was really on our radar in [region].*
>
> ***Interviewer:*** *I remember reading something about [region] being the lowest diagnosis rate in Scotland.*
>
> ***EP:*** *And I think at the moment we seem to have a spike in it, and I don't know – you know – where that's come from.*

The 'Witches Brew' of Actual Practice: Division, Normalisation and Psychiatric Knowledge

When discussing 'the problem of rationalities' in *Questions of Method*, Foucault (1991b, p. 81) highlights the roles of 'witches brew' in understanding the enactment of governmental rationalities. The term is used to describe the functioning of power at the micro level in overcoming resistance to its enactment through the various actions and enactments of the subjects in response to the resistance. The critical point was that power did not function according to an 'ideal', to official programmes or technologies, but as always unfolding within the limitations inherent within the 'actual' elements of the apparatus and through specific encounters with resistance and blockages to its functioning and flow. This critical point was elaborated and put to work by Brady (2011) in her study of enactment of Australian single-parent welfare reforms. Drawing on the work of Lipsky (2010), Brady's work highlighted the role of those involved in service delivery as not just about implementing policy, but as 'making it up', as creating discursive spaces within official rationalities where alternative discourses and rationalities would assist in the enactment of these 'official' rationalities. The work of Brady and Lipsky are relevant here: both consider the role of individual subjects within agencies functioning at the micro level of government in the fabrication of 'actual' practices within official governmental rationalities. The relevance of the 'witches brew' of actual practices to this project was made visible by the descriptions of what was considered to be 'intervention', but also in the use of psychiatric knowledge to construct 'complex' problems and the function this construction played in managing these problems.

As outlined earlier, both in the genealogical account but also in the official and professional account of the procedures of additional support needs, the image constructed is of a holistic, supportive and inclusive system that adapts the school environment to meet specific needs, with adaptations based on careful assessment of risk to learning. Additional needs were not considered fixed but fluid and 'fixable' through application of specific adjustments. The forms of knowledge present within the system allowed for structuring of problem explanations as 'caused' by attachment issues, trauma and/or disadvantage, with history and context considered central for understanding the problem. In this system, diagnosis and disorder were not required, support would be based on need, and additional provision would be provided to accommodate needs. However, despite the claims of inclusion of difference and adjustment of environment to meet this, descriptions of 'interventions' by educational professionals highlight the young person as the target, rather than the environment. In the following excerpt, a school teacher is describing a 'nurture group' intervention, explicitly describing young people as the target, with the aim being the development of 'regulation skills' in order for them to be able to 'go back to class'. The discourse of attachment and the importance of context are visible within this explanation of the 'problem', but despite this, young people remain the 'target' for intervention, with self-regulation the desired outcome:

> ***Teacher:*** *That's right – yeah. And obviously, particularly in our area and where we are, we've got to get that bit right for a lot of our kids before they're in a place to learn and look at – you know – other areas of the curriculum. So [name]*

runs a nurture group. And originally, we set that up and it supported about six children all morning. And what we found was that was really effective in giving them that intense, small group support, trying to teach them some of the regulation skills and strategies and – you know – lots of emotional work. And then they would be able to go back to class and they were beginning to graduate. The level of need increased if you like and what we had to do was change resource to have the nurture facility running three times a day for an hour and fifty minutes.

Teacher 2: *But there was more children who really felt were identifying that need – they were needing that wee bit of nurture for all sorts of reasons. Some of them were looked after and accommodated. Others – you know – we know were coming from challenging home backgrounds – there's some who've never learned 'no' – they've never learned. An adult saying when I mean 'no'... I mean no – there's a lot of children who haven't learned that self-regulation because when I kick off at home and I shout and scream and swear I eventually get what I want. So I'm going to try that in school, and all of a sudden, 'this isn't working; why's it not? – Ahh, I can't cope with this because it's so different to home.' So we now run the nurture three times a day, and that allows us to target just a few more children, and a bit more age-specific, too. So we've got like a senior nurture group –*

Another discontinuity between the 'official' procedures and the 'witches brew' was the role of psychiatric knowledge. As outlined earlier, the accounts of the grid presented an image of a system structured by discourse of attachment and trauma. Accordingly, problems would be considered holistically and contextualised by environment and development; within this reality, diagnosis was not considered to be required, with the knowledges and approaches available considered appropriate for the forms of 'problems' made visible. Despite this, psychiatric knowledge and discourse frequently appeared in descriptions of problems, appearing to be deployed to construct certain problems as severe and complex. In the first excerpt below, an educational psychologist is describing whole school and individual interventions as being structured by the discourse of attachment, but goes on to use psychiatric discourse when describing the specifics of the 'problem' presentation, which can be considered as opening up space for the deployment of either discourse when 'treating the problem'. In the second excerpt, a different educational psychologist offers an account of disadvantage in a school catchment area, connecting this to the complexity of the problems that have required additional support in a particular school; however, towards the end of the excerpt they highlight that provision for Autism Spectrum

Disorder (ASD) had been set up in the school because of the number of young people considered 'not to be managing'. This 'not managing' was attributed to being on the 'spectrum' despite the extensive description of contextual factors:

Excerpt 1:

Educational psychologist: *In general, as a service we have provided loads of training and intervention, either in a whole school or an individual basis around about supporting children who look as if they've got some kind of insecure attachment. And our schools – that's the language they speak. So if you're thinking about a child who was a bit dysregulated, who's got poor attention and concentration and they can't sit on their bum – are you thinking there's something intrinsically wrong with that child, or are you saying that developmentally they're actually younger than their chronological age.*

Excerpt 2:

Educational psychologist (2): *The Scottish government have provided funding to schools or local authorities who have schools within the most deprived areas of Scotland. And [school] doesn't fall within the most deprived area, but the level of need that it mops up is phenomenal. You know, some of the most bizarre and complex cases I've had, have come from [school].*

[...]

So [school] has a real – and again, I think looking more widely at the community, it's a community where we seem to be two, three, sometimes four generations being involved with families. You can make links back – oh, that's such-and-such's grandchild, or that's so-and-so's great aunty.

[...]

There's areas in [catchment area of school] that were used as kind of – I don't like to say 'dumping ground', but that's essentially what they were. You know, they moved out the really difficult families from those difficult challenged areas in [city], and they wanted to bring them out to the countryside. So they brought them to places like [catchment area of school]. But – you know – the sensible person in you goes 'well, actually, they've just brought

> *the problems with them'. So we've got generational issues with – you know – families who've never worked, who've always been on benefits – you know – repeated histories of abuse of various forms, substance misuse, all that kind of stuff. So [school] is our new melting pot of all of that, and has some really challenging kids. But has historically had a really good reputation within the authority, as being a school that just manages and gets on with – you know – and the course of time that I've had that school, we've set up an ASD-specific provision, because we had a real spike of kids that were just not managing because they were on the spectrum.*

The reality of additional support needs constructed through actual practices at the level of the individual professionals within schools highlights the continued functioning of psychiatric knowledge in the construction and management of problems considered to be complex, despite claims of accommodating individual needs through school and curriculum adjustment. The system, rather than being inclusive of need and adjusting to meet these, appears to function through division of young people into levels of severity and application of 'interventions' as a means of shaping them to fit school, rather than the other way around. At the lower levels of the staged approach, problems are constructed by attachment or trauma with intervention at the level of the school, with support from educational psychology. However, as the 'problem' is moved up the staged system, it moves into a discursive space where it can become reconstituted by psychiatric knowledge and discourse, allowing for targeting by psychiatric intervention.

The reconstituting by psychiatric knowledge appears to be legitimated by the concept of 'underlying abnormality' being applied to 'problems' that are not resolved through school-based approaches. In the following accounts by two different educational psychologists, the process of division is visible; in the first account ADHD becomes a potential explanation if the problem persists once attachment or contextual factors have been considered. Similarly, in the second account, ADHD appears to exist alongside attachment to explain why the young person is unable to 'keep their bum on the seat' despite attachment 'work' having been conducted by the previous case holder. In both accounts, what appears to be made visible is a line across which 'problems' cross to become assigned to a different form of knowledge for explanation and, thus, for alternative forms of intervention. The reality created appears to be a reconstituted continuum of need divided into a normal and abnormal binary. On one side are problems of less severity, manageable within the apparatus of education, and on the other side are complex and severe problems underpinned by abnormality and requiring specialist psychiatric consideration. In both cases, ADHD becomes a potential alternative explanation, allowing the young person to become a target for 'treatment' with psycho-stimulant medication:

Excerpt 1:

Educational psychologist: *Well, the assessment would be information from the school, gathering information from parents – you know – developmental – general developmental history is something that we – you know – really blindingly obvious or is there nothing. And covering things like divorce and separation. Trying to rule out is this an attachment difficulty. And then if you're coming down on the side of it being ADHD or a neuro-developmental difficulty, in terms of intervention, I don't know that we've got a – it's probably an area where we don't have a huge amount of resource.*

Excerpt 2:

Educational psychologist (2): *I think historically, as a service, we've had more of a focus on attachment and trauma. And that was kind of coming from the top down. You know, [name] and [name] and [name] – so the three previous principals that we've had – that was very much their focus and their area of expertise, their area of interest.*

[…]

When [name] was off sick earlier on this year, I picked up a case from her where she said 'actually, I think it's both – I think we've got attachment things going on but actually they can't keep their bum on the seat and – you know – I think they've just been really unlucky – they've got a double whammy'.

Avoiding the Inscription of 'Severity' as 'Real' Difference

In her examination of the means by which young people were subject to governance through educational policy and practice, Watson (2010) highlights how 'mainstreaming difference' through the discourse of inclusion does not result in the reduction in the use of diagnostic labels; rather the use of the technology increases and its use changes. The critical point illuminated by Watson's analysis was visible across the various conversations with educational professionals conducted for this project: that psychiatric diagnosis become a resource for the production of forms of subjectivity, allowing governance of the subject through associated technologies and expertise. The continued role for psychiatric knowledge was visible in the process of division and normalisation that structured the actual practices of additional support needs at the micro level of their application: without the continued role of the knowledge, the problems considered severe would remain within the mainstream school and would require intervention to reduce the risk to future learning. This continued availability of psychiatric knowledge and associated technologies allows for division and reconstitution of problems as severe and complex and as requiring psychiatric expertise and input, allowing for schools to incorporate new forms of management alongside those within the apparatus of education.

An additional critical point that will be offered as part of this analysis, however, relates to the work of Lipsky (2010), drawn on earlier in the chapter. In his analysis, the actual practices at the micro level of governmental rationalities were shaped by multiple competing requirements and influences, including inadequate resources, growing demand for services, vague policy requirements and goals, etc. In the present analysis, all of the above competing requirements and influences were visible in the apparatus of education – made possible by the intersecting discourses of social inclusion and additional support needs – exerting pressure on the individual subjects enacting the practices of governance. These are visible in two main themes that were repeated across all conversations with educational professionals: the reconstitution of local council educational services according to changing budgetary requirements, and the changing role of educational psychology from a direct therapeutic service to a 'consultation model' due to reduced capacity and increased demand. When considered against this background, the application of 'underlying abnormality' to 'problems' not resolved through school-based approaches can be considered to be a fabrication of practice in response to the problem's resistance to intervention. However, rather than the resistance to 'treatment' being underpinned by 'severity' or 'complexity' caused by a biomedical abnormality, this can be considered a response to normalisation occurring instead of structural change, placed upon the apparatus of education by the increased demands conditioned by the requirement for inclusion and for mainstream school to meet the needs of *every* young person.

Chapter 5: Part 1

Fixing the ADHD Child: The Clinical Case File

The following chapter provides a description of the analysis of the clinical case notes of several young people who had received a diagnosis of ADHD. Those who agreed to take part in the project were not pre-selected for the project, but were the young people attending appointment during the periods in which I was embedded within the service and who consented to take part in the project. Some of the young people who allowed access to their case notes had been involved with the service for several years, others several months. This time period was particularly useful, as it provided access to a changing background of arguments and logics in relation to the 'problem' of young people within the service. Over the years covered by the case files, it was possible to detect various 'truths, explanations, categorisations and taxonomies, vocabularies and diagnoses' (Rose, 1996, p. 25) at work in the problematisation of young people, allowing for an examination of the ways the 'truths' that structured the explanations contained in the case files had come to be formed.

In total, I accessed 10 sets of clinical case files, with all of the files representing males; as mentioned, this was not pre-selection, but a representation of the gender of young people attending the Child and Adolescent Mental Health Service (CAMHS) for ADHD-related clinical appointments. The dominance of the male gender constituting the overall number receiving the diagnosis is a well-documented contradiction in the neurodevelopmental explanation of ADHD: according to its own frame of reference, if ADHD is neurodevelopmental in origin, the spread of diagnosis should be equal across both genders, but this is not the case, with the ratio of males to females receiving the diagnosis ranging from 2:1 to 9:1 (see: Biederman, Faraone, Monuteaux, Bober, & Cadogen, 2004).

In addition to the case files, I was also able to access several years of CAMHS management team meeting minutes. These documents provided access to the various policies and political trends impacting on the service, which was particularly useful in providing the discursive context for the changing clinical procedures documented in the case notes. The procedure followed for processing the textual material was based upon what I have termed 'layering': simultaneous reading and analysis within and across case notes, meeting minutes and relevant policies discovered through analysis of the team meeting minutes. When 'layered' together, the textual material can be considered to have provided the discursive background that made possible what was sayable and doable within the service. Within this background, it was possible to locate the 'truths' that had come to form the problematisation of conduct; the forms of specialist knowledge and skills deployed in diagnosing and intervening in problematised conduct; the sites in which the conduct was judged, assessed, evaluated, understood, and acted upon; and the interacting conditions that allowed the 'contemporary matrix' and its 'diverse and contradictory logics' (Rose, 1996, p. 24), to condition what was sayable and doable within the service at this moment in time.

Despite being positioned as Chapter 5 in the overall document, the steps outlined here are the starting point for the entire project, with the process of 'working backwards' described in the methodological plan commencing from the 'problems and solutions' discovered during the analysis that underpins this chapter. The analysis was conducted in two stages: the starting point was a detailed analysis of the problems and explanations that constructed the initial referral letters for each of the young people represented by the case notes. This was followed by an analysis of the different ways the 'problem' in the referral letter was constructed within the service and what 'treatment' these constructions legitimated. What I discovered through this stage was a changing discursive background, one the shifted from coexistence of a multiplicity of explanations and idiosyncratic procedures to a dominance of psychiatric discourse and a formulised 'approach' legitimated by the problems it solved. The second stage of the analysis aimed to reveal what made it possible for this dominance to occur. Through analysis of the 'treatments' outlined in the case notes and simultaneous analysis of the meeting minutes, the appearance of a detailed 'approach' for the management of ADHD referrals was detected. The appearance of this approach at the particular historical juncture at which it appeared was critical in conditioning the possibility for the eventual dominance of psychiatric discourse within the service, but also beyond the service in the local schools. The analysis of what made it possible for this dominance to occur consisted of deconstructing the statements at work in the legitimation of the approach within the meeting minutes and reconnecting these to the wider policies, discourses and events that allowed for the legitimating statements to be in the 'true' at the point in time at which they were uttered. The aim of the analysis was to locate the statements that constructed the ADHD approach and track their appearance from within the service to the discursive formations that provided the invisible lines of authority upon which the procedures were legitimated.

A final point to make regarding the 'working backwards' approach is that the analysis in this chapter allowed me to locate the 'problem' of increased referrals from educational establishments and its role in conditioning the possibility of the ADHD approach that aided the eventual dominance of psychiatric discourse and practice. This analytical point provided the starting point from which to 'work backwards' in the previous chapter. This working backwards across the shifting discursive realities of health and educations sites highlights how they are undeniably linked in the construction of young people as 'having' ADHD: the problem of 'additional support needs' discussed in the last chapter can be seen to have created the conditions for increased referrals from educational establishments to CAMHS – the very problem the ADHD 'approach' was proposed to solve.

The procedure within the 'approach' that would solve the problem of increased referrals was to 'work' directly with schools to provide support to manage ADHD within educational sites. However, rather than reduce referrals to CAMHS, the 'approach' can be seen to have conditioned the possibility for ADHD as an explanation to increase in dominance within educational establishments, creating a mutually reinforcing discursive process that resulted in the proliferation of ADHD diagnosis and treatment.

Constructing the Problem: Analysis of Referral Reasons

ADHD is very much an object of psychiatric knowledge and discourse, appearing in various forms since in emergence in its contemporary iteration in the *DSM-III*. When considering ADHD at the level of the clinical files, however, it became apparent that a diagnosis of ADHD was not solely the result of the deployment of psychiatric knowledge by psychiatrists. There were case files that highlighted the fixing of ADHD solely by psychiatric knowledge and discourse, but the majority of the case files (7) highlighted ADHD as an eventual outcome, as something that gradually emerged from within a multitude of competing explanations, with a range of non-psychiatric professionals involved in constructing the problem in different ways prior to ADHD being fixed in place. In each of these case files, the 'problem' that resulted in the young person being referred to the service was constructed by explanations other than ADHD. For example, one of the explanations for the 'problem' that led to the young person being referred can be considered to be constructed by an 'attachment' discourse:

> [Mother] has advised that she has suffered episodes of anxiety throughout her life. Her pregnancy with [young person] was unexpected and precipitated her setting up a household with [new partner]. This was a very anxious time for her. She conceived again shortly after [young person]'s birth and her daughter [child] was born 11 months after [young person]. Following this, [mother] suffered from post-natal depression. She believes this impaired her emotional availability for both children.

The above excerpt, whilst not stating attachment explicitly, includes the statement 'impaired emotional availability', positioning this as something that should have been provided by the mother but which was disrupted by post-natal depression. When constructed by an attachment discourse, problems are positioned as resulting from a lack of containing secure caregiving experience disrupting the quality of the child–parent dyad (see: Brumariu, 2015; Cassidy, 1994). According to this explanation, the parent–child relationship is the foundation of secure attachment relationships and it is upon this foundation that personality and future well-being is built, with those considered to be securely attached more able to 'self-regulate' how they react to the wider world around them. In other files, attachment as explanation was more explicit:

> Given the developmental history, I think that many of [young person]'s difficulties stem from an insecure anxious attachment and are compounded by [mother]'s diffidence in parenting him.

In both of these accounts, implicitly and explicitly, the difficulties are constructed as the result of an impaired caregiving dyad, with the resulting 'impaired emotion regulation' or 'insecure anxious attachment' considered to be the cause of the problem requiring assessment by mental health services. By constructing the problem as a problem of attachment, the ability to regulate emotion is positioned as an attribute, one that is learned within the caregiving experience, and which provides those who have gained the skill with an ability to regulate the impact of their emotions on their behaviour and environment. The opposite position in this explanation, and the one that can be considered to be implicit in the problem constructions located in the case files, is that emotion 'dysregulation' is the outcome of the poor early attachment experience, which has resulted in the young person being unable to 'manage' their behaviours and emotions.

A further explanation located in the referral reasons emphasised the impact on the development of the young person of a variety of negative social events and circumstances. This appeared in different forms; for example, as the result of domestic violence (first excerpt) or as part of a collection of multiple interacting stressors (second excerpt):

> **Excerpt 1:**
>
> *My impression was that the family had experienced a number of difficulties that may have made providing consequences difficult. Paternal alcohol use and domestic violence coupled with maternal depression may have influenced the development of the current situation.*
>
> **Excerpt 2:**
>
> *[Father] caused serious injury to his child and received a prison sentence. He was released from prison and placed on licence for three years on condition he was not to have unsupervised contact. [Mother and father]'s mental health was also an issue and alcohol use and honesty around the amount being consumed, affecting their ability to address problems. There was an overdose attempt by [father] when [young person] was in the house, leading to concerns about the impact on his wellbeing. There were also concerns around [young person]'s school attendance with [mother] colluding*

> *with him on this and the chaotic household with a number of adults in and out the family home. It is concluded that [young person] has experienced physical and emotional abuse and has impacted on his mental health.*

In both explanations, the problem is positioned as resulting from an interaction between environmental factors, such as negative social events and circumstances, impacting on the normative development of skills, abilities and attributes. In this problem construction, negative social events and circumstances are positioned as 'risk factors' – a 'thing' in the young person's context considered to be detrimental to positive developmental outcomes (see: Walker et al., 2007). In this account, commonly accepted psychological attributes, such as behaviour, cognition, emotion, etc., are considered to be individual outcomes of naturally occurring developmental processes that are entwined with multiple, interrelated contexts or systems within which we grow, including family, school, peers and communities. In this account, development is divided into a 'typical' and 'atypical' binary, with each outcome dependent on the presence or not of risk factors at various developmental stages. In both excerpts above, the role of 'parenting' is present, with its absence or diminished capacity constructed as resulting in a lack of behavioural consequences for bad behaviour or behaviour problems not being addressed at all. In these explanations, the referral problem is constructed as resulting from the interaction of 'poor parenting' with the young person's normative developmental processes, with mental health problems positioned as the outcome of this interaction.

As well as accounts that constructed the problem as something that had developed, there were also explanations where a number of 'symptoms', or ADHD as disorder, were offered as explanations for the problematic behaviours:

Excerpt 1:

> *[Young person] is active and aggressive. He is biting and spitting. In the clinic-room today he would not sit still and take 'no' for an answer. I understand he is on level 3 staged intervention and is likely to require additional support in school, however his cognitive abilities appear to be normal. I think [young person] will need further consideration of possible attention deficit hyperactivity disorder and perhaps other conditions.*

Excerpt 2:

> *[Young person] displays hyperactivity, inattention and a degree of impulsiveness over all settings. [Mother] notes that [young person]'s school work has appeared disorganised in the past year and he seems to be struggling with his attention more than he has previously. Sleep has been a significant*

> *concern for some time and it sounds like [young person] can stay up until the early hours of the morning and get by on very little sleep the next day. [Young person] is also picky with his food and tends to graze on small amounts. [Young person]'s parents note that he appears isolated socially having no close friends and showing very little interest in developing peer relationships. I am going to request information on [young person]'s presentation at school as well as asking for any relevant correspondence, reports or assessments.*

In both statements, behavioural expression is positioned as representing the 'symptoms' of ADHD, with the disorder positioned as the explanation for the symptoms. These explanations can be considered to be constructed by psychiatric discourse; in these accounts, problem behaviours are positioned as 'symptoms' and as manifested by an abnormal endogenous process. The functioning of diagnosis in this explanation signifies that a process of assessment, interpretation and identification of the nature of the illness has been conducted by a qualified medical professional. The 'illness' diagnosed is positioned as the underlying cause of the symptoms, with the diagnosis arrived at through careful comparison of assessment information with medical disorder classification systems such as, in the case of ADHD, the *Diagnostic and Statistical Manual of Mental Disorders* or the *International Classification of Mental and Behavioural Disorders*.

The Diverse Logics of Problematisation

The various explanations within the clinical files, represented in the excerpts above, can be considered to be constructed upon two competing logics: one of development and one of abnormality. Both of these logics permeate the wider positivist research literature, underpinning psychological and psychiatric accounts respectively. A cursory glance at examples of the positivist literature regarding ADHD highlights the visibility of these competing knowledges and their distinctive logics. For example, Hellmer and Nyström (2017) position dysfunction at a neurochemical level, citing specific abnormally functioning neurotransmitters as indicative of a genetic level vulnerability which results in the expression of ADHD. The logic of abnormality contained within this example exemplifies the wider psychiatric explanation of ADHD: problematic behaviours are positioned as symptoms of neurotransmitter dysregulation, genetic anomalies, and defects in brain structure and function. In these accounts, ADHD is constructed as ontologically distinct from normative social behaviours, as a deviation from normal human biological expression and as a result of disordered biochemical or neurophysiological processes. The biomedical 'treatment' with psychotropic medication that is authorised by this problematisation is presented as correcting the biomedical or neurophysiological imbalances considered to underpin the disorder, with psychostimulant drugs, such as methylphenidate, considered to reduce 'synaptic concentration of norepinephrine and dopamine' in different brain regions. The outcomes considered to result from the psychotropic medication are improved attention, enhanced task-specific focus and reduced distractibility and impulsivity.

In contrast to psychiatric discourse and the logic of abnormality, Brocki, Forslund, Frick, and Bohlin (2017) position 'self-regulation' as important in the 'development' of ADHD. The authors claim the individual attributes of 'emotion regulation' and 'cognitive regulation' as connected to ADHD, with early developmental experiences positioned as influential in the development of these attributes. In this account, problematic early experience and its impact on the development of these key individual attributes are positioned as increasing the risk for later development of ADHD. The logic of development visible in this example constructs problematic behaviour not as abnormality but as maladaptation, with maladaptation represented as an outcome of the adaptation of the developmental processes to social context. Within a developmental logic of maladaptation, development is constructed as an adaptive, multi-process system, with the various processes occurring across multiple levels of context. In this account, young people are constructed as complex living systems that interact effectively and ineffectively over time with the various contexts in which they are embedded. Problematic behaviours as maladaptation are represented as continuous to normative behavioural expression, which is in contrast to the differentiation of problematic behaviour from normal behavioural expression by biomedical discourse, with problematic behaviour considered a symptom of an underlying abnormality (see: Cicchetti, 2016).

Discontinuity of Practice: Comparing CAMHS Practice with Official Knowledge

Despite the two logics visible in the referral problems, and in the examples of 'official' knowledge above, seemingly contradictory of each other, both have become entwined within the discourse and practice of 'developmental psychopathology'. This was a particularly important point within this project because a contrasting position was discovered within the case notes and more widely within the discourse and practice of the service. Arguably, developmental psychopathology has become an increasingly dominant form of official knowledge within the institutions of child and adolescent mental health, with its emergence associated with the coalescing of distinct institutional knowledges, including behavioural genetics, neuroscience, psychiatry, and developmental psychology, around the problem of 'at-risk' children and young people. Over the last 20–30 years, the discourse and practice of young people's mental health can be seen to have become integrative and, rather than competing over explanation, the various disciplinary knowledges can be seen to have combined, with problem explanations becoming more expansive, incorporating more and more domains of the young person's experiences and environment. An example of the combined logics within the discourse of developmental psychopathology is visible in the following excerpt from an 'official' knowledge source – a journal article. In the excerpt, 'abnormality' remains but takes the form of 'neurophysiological associates of disorder'. It is no longer positioned as a cause, however, but as a marker, as an underlying abnormality that will only find expression through a dynamic interactive developmental process:

> So important is the perspective of development for understanding psychopathology that it spawned a new discipline—'developmental psychopathology'—which has seen remarkable advances since its introduction but has yet to completely fulfil its promise. To do this requires maintaining a thoroughgoing developmental perspective. When development is taken seriously, there are implications for how to understand psychopathology, describe and conceptualize the origins and course of disorder, and interpret research findings. From this perspective, disorders are complex products of development; for example, neurophysiological associates of disorder can be viewed not as causes but as markers, the development of which needs to be understood. Research on developmental psychopathology requires an examination of the history of problem behavior from early in life, and it unites multiple features of adaptation and maladaptation (contextual, experiential, physiological, and genetic). (Sroufe, 2009)

In this expanded discourse of mental health, problematic behaviours are positioned as the result of 'bidirectional interactions' occurring within and across genetic, neural, behavioural and environmental levels of human context. The new combined logic is one of development but within a biomedical framework, neatly summarised by the concept of 'probabilistic epigenesis' that constructs the description of gene and environment interaction at the core of the above statement. In this new logic, genes are positioned as initiating developmental pathways that are receptive to influences from the cellular to the social contextual level, with problematic behaviour represented as the result of 'coaction', 'transaction' and 'interaction' across the multiple levels of human context. The entwinement of these competing logics allows for the construction of an infinite number of events as 'risk factors' that contribute to an increased likelihood of the development of problematic behaviours and the categorisation of both social context and individual behavioural expression as the target of intervention (see: Gottlieb, 2007).

Within this new framework of understanding, ADHD is positioned as the result of 'coaction', 'transaction' and 'interaction' of faulty genes with multiple environmental risk factors which, over time, interact bi-directionally, creating individual trajectories towards the disordered outcome; the behaviour becomes a target of biomedical treatment, with known 'risk factors' such as parenting approaches, school systems and dysfunctional household also considered valid targets of the 'heterogeneous 'psy' judgements' of ancillary clinical and non-clinical professionals that constitute the network of professionals that target what are represented as 'mental health conditions'. Despite the growing prominence of this new discursive formation of mental health within official knowledge and practice, it was not visible in discourse and practice of the CAMHS service. This was indicated to me by a discontinuity between what is represented in official knowledges and what was represented by the case notes. Within official knowledges, there is a clear shift from coexistence to the merging of the logics of development and abnormality, whereas over the several years covered by the case files, the opposite was detected: that there was a shift from coexistence of the logics to a dominance of the biomedical logic and psychiatric discourse.

This eventual dominance of the biomedical logic was visible in the case notes of the young people who had been involved with the service over several years. In the older case notes, when compared to the more recent case notes, the diagnosis of ADHD was an eventual outcome of multiple assessments, with several different explanations offered prior to ADHD emerging as the explanation for the behaviour. In the more recent case files, problems are immediately fixed as an expression of ADHD, with no alternative explanations visible in the case notes. This was also evident in letters from general practitioners requesting assessment of the behaviour of young people: in the clinical files of young people who had been involved with the service over several years, referral letters described difficulties in general terms and requested non-specific assessment, whereas more recent referral letters constructed the difficulties as ADHD, requesting specific ADHD assessment.

Excerpt 1:

> *I should welcome your assessment of the above young boy. He is reported to be an extremely destructive and angry young child. I understand he is in primary 2 at [school]. He struggles to make friends, appears very solitary and at time insecure. His mum is becoming increasingly concerned regarding his behaviour, and accordingly I should welcome your formal assessment.*

Excerpt 2:

> *I would be grateful for your assessment of this seven-year-old boy. His mother is single and is struggling to manage the behaviour of the boy who is on the go all day and who was unable to sit still for a minute in the clinic setting.*
>
> *[Young person] appears to have average intelligence. He has good imaginative play, understands language and has age-appropriate pencil skills. However, he is constantly in trouble at school and demonstrated oppositional and defiant behaviour to his mother today.*

> *I think mum needs a great deal of support with behavioural management but I also feel that his activity levels and attention span may be consistent with a diagnosis of ADHD and I would be interested in your formal assessment of such.*

Shifting Procedures: From Clinical Judgement to Streamlined Assessment

This shifting logic constructing the problematisation of young people within the service reveals a discontinuity with formalised institutional knowledges and practice of young people's mental health. Given the historical coexistence of the logics and recent entwinement in the discourse and practice of developmental psychopathology, the dominance of a logic of abnormality was unusual and in contrast to official accounts of young people's mental health. Through layering the case notes and the minutes of the management team meetings, I was able to connect the shifting logics and wider discursive background in the service with the emergence of an approach to the diagnosis and treatment of ADHD that I have termed the 'ADHD machine'. I have changed the official title of the approach to keep the service anonymous in order to protect the identity of the young people who allowed access their case notes and clinical appointments.

The role of machine in shaping the discursive background within the service was made visible through an increasing frequency of statements regarding the machine in the minutes and a corresponding increase in frequency of statements connected to the discourse of psychiatry in the case files. Statements regarding the ADHD machine emerge in the management team meetings from late 2003 and continued until 2008. Correspondingly, over the same period in the clinical files, there was an increase in statements connected to the logic of abnormality and the biomedical understanding of ADHD. There was also an increased 'formalisation' of approach, with differing individual clinical approaches and judgement gradually being replaced by a formulaic approach comprised of questionnaires, child observations, and clinical interviews of parents and teachers.

The questionnaires were an important element in this new procedure and in the eventual dominance of the biomedical logic – prior to the machine, individual clinical judgement allowed for multiple explanations, but replacement with psychometrics, such as the 'revised Tanner-Whitehouse questionnaire' and the 'Conners' rating scales, replaced individual clinical judgement with the objects of psychiatric knowledge constructed by the questionnaires. These constructs – hyperactivity, inattention, concentration – can be considered to have gained their legitimacy over clinical judgement through a rhetorical warranting by the concepts of validity, reliability and objectivity associated with psychometrics. Procedurally, however, the psychometric assessment performed a function in 'solving' the problem being 'assessed' through the quantification, comparison and differentiation from an imaginary 'norm'. The use of this psychometric assessment can be considered to create the image of the procedures of diagnosis outlined above. However, rather than locating a 'real' illness, their constructs are fixed on the young person through application of a normal/abnormal cut-off, allowing for deployment of 'underlying disorder' as explanation for the abnormality they have constructed.

A final shift in procedure was detected beyond 2008, with the ADHD machine gradually being replaced by what was described as a 'streamlined assessment' process. This new approach was what I observed in the clinical appointments. During the sessions, the procedure consisted of the administering of a 'service-developed', biomedically informed, 'ADHD care package clinic documentation' proforma. The new streamlined approach replaced the application of various psychometric assessments with one 'proforma' containing several questions regarding 'clinical presentation', 'side effects and medication issues' and 'comorbid disorders'. The output from the new approach was quantified as an 'inattention total score' and a 'hyperactivity/impulsivity total score'.

Chapter 5: Part 2

The Problems It Solved: Deconstructing the Legitimacy of the Machine

The description of the machine within the minutes constructed it as a 'nurse-led', 'multi-disciplinary approach', consisting of 'nursing', 'psychology' and a 'teacher'. The procedure was positioned as unique in its approach to solving the problem of ADHD as responsibility for diagnosis and prescription would move from psychiatrists to an 'advanced nurse practitioner' with specialist skills in 'nurse prescribing'. By moving responsibility for ADHD to an advanced nurse practitioner with specialist skills in prescribing, the machine would allow for a fast-tracked ADHD referral process that would allow for increased efficiency in diagnosis and prescription of psychostimulant medication. The involvement of a teacher legitimated integration with schools, warranting 'support' and school-based intervention to be offered to schools alongside psychostimulant medication.

The first appearance of statements regarding the machine was in a draft 'CAMHS service specification', which was developed to communicate the 'aims and philosophy' of the 'new' service after its 'launch' as the Child and Adolescent Mental Health Service. However, the service had a longer history than was revealed in the minutes, a history that was made available to me in the conversations I had during my time embedded in the service: prior to its launch as CAMHS, two separate services – a Child Psychology service and Child Psychiatry service – inhabited the same building. It was the merging of these two distinct services that underpinned the launch, with reconstitution of the two services as CAMHS, a requirement of an emerging policy requirement for 'integrated services' and 'partnership working' across children's services. The appearance of the ADHD machine at this juncture corresponded with several problems impacting on the newly integrated service. At various locations across the minutes, the machine is positioned as an answer to 'increased demands on caseloads', 'increased wait times for initial assessment appointment', 'increased school referrals' and 'to improve assessment, management and liaison with schools for children with ADHD'.

The procedures of the ADHD machine described above played an important role in conditioning the eventual dominance of the biomedical logic. Through moving problems to single clinician contact within the service and fast-tracking through a biomedically structured assessment process, the procedure can be considered as simultaneously closing down non-biomedical ways of constructing problems referred to the service at the same time as allowing for a proliferation of biomedical and psychiatric statements. The movement of responsibility for assessment to a single clinician was made possible through the 'problem of demand' being constructed as 'caseloads being filled with assessments for problem behaviours often represented as ADHD'. By moving to a single point of contact, the machine was positioned as able to increase the capacity of the remaining clinicians and, thus, as reducing the 'risk to young people with other mental health problems, such as depression, anorexia or suicidality' waiting too long for assessment and intervention.

The association of 'risk' with increased time waiting for intervention can be considered to connect to a biomedical account of early intervention, where intervening early in the problem cycle is considered to prevent lasting consequences through treatment reducing the problem before it becomes intractable (see: Early Intervention Foundation, 2015). The early intervention discourse can also be considered to offer legitimacy to the proposal of fast-tracked assessment, diagnosis and treatment and liaison with schools. Both procedural elements, considered through an early intervention discourse, suggest increased efficiency in the detection, diagnosis and treatment of ADHD within CAMHS and across schools, with the efficiency allowing detection and treatment before it increases in severity.

Rather than solving the problem of demand, however, reducing the number of clinicians authorised to offer clinical judgement can be considered to have closed down the possibility of statements outside of the psychiatric explanation of ADHD informing the assessment process of young people referred to the service. Prior to the emergence of the machine, statements outside of the ADHD explanation are present within the case files, whereas beyond the emergence of the machine, alternative explanations gradually disappear, replaced by biomedical and psychiatric statements. An important element in this eventuality was the reduction of CAMHS contact points to one single clinician, but also the replacing of their 'clinical judgement' with a formulaic assessment process comprised of 'objective measures of ADHD'. The questionnaires that were deployed required parents and teachers to rate the frequency of hyperactive, inattentive and/or impulsive behaviours occurring in the young person as well as document challenging behaviours and school-based problems. These questionnaires displayed an increasing visibility in the case notes over time, but importantly the constructs of the questionnaires displayed an increasing visibility in the handwritten case notes and various letters sent to referring professionals, thus extending the explanation beyond the service into the wider network of children's services.

The underlying subscales of the dominant questionnaire within this process is considered to measure the presence of oppositional behaviour, cognitive problems/inattention, hyperactivity and global ADHD, with the parent or teacher rating the presence of the problem behaviours presented by the questions as 'not true at all', 'just a little true', 'pretty much true' or 'very much true'. The questions asked include (taken from the Connors' rating scale):

(1) *Inattentive, easily distracted?*
(2) *Defiant?*
(3) *Restless in the 'squirmy' sense?*

(4) *Forgets things he/she has already learned?*
(5) *Disturbs other children?*
(6) *Actively defies or refuses to comply with adults' requests?*
(7) *Is always 'on the go' or acts as if driven by a motor?*
(8) *Poor in spelling?*
(9) *Cannot remain still?*
(10) *Spiteful or vindictive?*

However, rather than indicating the presence of a naturally occurring phenomena, such as oppositionality, cognitive problems, inattention, hyperactivity or ADHD, the questionnaires can be considered to construct the ADHD child by problematising young people through biomedical logic: the questionnaires assume that the symptoms indicate the presence of the underlying abnormality considered to cause the symptoms. As such, the behaviours being considered can only be framed through the lens that informs the questions – 'inattentive', 'spiteful', 'vindictive', 'easily distracted', 'defiant', 'can't sit still', etc. – and the view of the subject answering the questions is equally shaped by the questions asked. Despite the quantification process (not true at all, just a little true, pretty much true, very much true), and the behavioural characteristics quantified, being vague and difficult to define, the rhetorical objectivity bestowed by positive scientific concepts such as 'psychometric properties', 'validity' and 'reliability' transforms the subjective nature of the responses into objective factual 'hard data' about the young person.

The Expanding Authority of Nursing: Advanced Nurse Practitioner

An important element through which the ADHD machine gained dominance can be connected to the positions of 'advanced nurse practitioner' and 'nurse prescriber'. Historically, in the service, ADHD assessment, diagnosis and prescription of psychostimulant medication had been the remit of consultant child psychiatrists; however, moving responsibility away from psychiatry to nursing was legitimated upon the clinician being an 'advanced nurse practitioner' who was able to 'prescribe' psychostimulant medication as intervention. The emergence of these new roles of nursing is important to contextualise as they functioned as key elements in legitimating movement of responsibility for ADHD within the service, but also as key procedural components of the everyday enactment of the procedures of the machine.

A consideration of nursing literature highlights the emergence of 'advanced nurse practitioner' and 'nurse prescriber' in nursing discourse and practice from mid-1990 onwards. The training programmes that converted nursing staff to advanced nurse practitioners appeared in the early 1990s, with the role appearing in Primary Care settings around the same time. Completing training bestowed the title of advanced nurse practitioner, allowing individual nurses to 'receive patients with undifferentiated and undiagnosed problems and make an assessment of their health-care needs, based on highly-developed nursing knowledge and skills' and 'make differential diagnoses using decision-making and problem-solving skills'. Similarly, the emergence of the position of nurse prescriber appears in nursing discourse and practice around the same time as the advanced nurse practitioner. Like the advanced nurse practitioner, for individual nurses to have authority to prescribe, they were required to undertake training before receiving the title. Initially, those who held the title had limited prescribing authority, but more recently the role has been bestowed with 'virtually the same independent prescribing powers as doctors' (see: Carnwell & Daly, 2003; Royal College of Nursing, 2012).

Both of these new nursing roles, and the training programmes that were considered to provide their skills and attributes, were conditioned by the requirements of a variety of health policies and reforms appearing in mid-to-late 1990s (see: Department of Health, 1997, 1999, 2000). A new requirement of this shifting policy background was the provision of locally informed, quick and reliable health care by local health-care professionals. This new approach was to be achieved through decentralisation of health-care provision to new partnerships between local councils and local health boards. In this local approach to health-care provision, local professionals were positioned as being in the best position to shape local service delivery through an awareness of local need. However, the new requirement for quick and reliable health care at a regional level, driven by local professionals, legitimated claims that health-care professionals would be required to increase efficiency and improve performance through a process of continual self-development and expansion of professional remit into areas normally performed by other professional groups.

To encourage this new requirement of continued self-directed improvement, new individual forms of governance were placed upon health-care professionals in order to achieve pay enhancement. The new individual governance framework replaced collective bargaining by labour unions with a series of 'national pay spines' and a competency-based career framework (KSF) (see: Buchan & Evans, 2007). This new salary framework removed salary enhancement from a process of collective bargaining, repositioning this as a requirement of individual professionals and only achievable through completing additional training, acquiring new skills or expanding professional remit to cover new areas of practice. Legitimated as the 'modernisation of NHS pay to reward career progressions', the new pay structure can be considered to function as a technology of governmental power, one that directed individual professionals towards self-enhancement and increased professional responsibility in order to meet the new requirements of locally driven health-care service needs.

The Intersecting Lines of the Well-being Agenda and Neoliberalism as Governance

The new requirements of health care that authorised the extension of the role of nursing discussed above can be seen to have emerged from within a shifting health policy context that marked the change of UK government in 1997. With the election of Labour in 1997, the NHS was subjected to a plethora of policies and reforms – most notably, the New NHS, Modern and Dependable, Making a Difference, and the NHS Plan. However, reform of the NHS in the period of the prior Conservative government from 1979 to 1997 was equally as legion, with several policies, and the shifts in practice they authorised, conditioning the possibility for the 'modernising' agenda constructed across the three policies referred to above. The strategies and technologies adopted by each administration differed, but each can be considered to be structured by the same politico-economic rationality – neoliberalism.

Typically, the concept of neoliberalism is considered to represent a drive for devolution and dispersal of state-provided roles to arms-length quasi-governmental agencies, an extension of market relationships into these and other aspects of society and an overarching aim of rolling back the state's involvement in the provision of these roles and services (see: Larner, 2000; Pownall, 2013). In earlier policies, the enactment of neoliberalism within the NHS takes the form of defunding services alongside the introduction of technologies of marketisation, including the creation and measurement of performance indicators, a requirement for discipline and economy in resource allocation and a shift to the promotion of competition in the provision of public services. Whereas, in post-1997 policies, the technologies of its enactment shift, taking the form of the codification of inter-agency working, increasing efficiency though governing staff towards self-improvement, and the targeting of the population through a 'public health' strategy aimed at encouraging 'well-being improvement strategies'. The emergence of well-being in the post-1997 policies marks an important shift in the functioning of neoliberalism, one that can be considered to have played an important role in conditioning the emergence of the ADHD machine through its legitimation as an approach able to promote well-being by intervening within health services and schools.

As outlined in Chapter 2, this project has been inspired by Foucauldian governmentality studies, which conceptualise neoliberalism as the means by which populations are governed as individuals at the micro-level through individual subjectivity and behaviour. From this perspective, critical consideration needs to move from political-economic accounts, as in the account above, towards a consideration of diffuse strategies (often legitimated by these policies) for knowing and shaping the actions and thoughts of the populace at the level of the individual subject. As Larner (2000) discusses, these ways of thinking are found in diverse realms, such as the workplace, educational institutions and health and welfare agencies, with all encouraging the human subject to see the self as an individualised and active subject and as responsible for the enhancement of well-being through 'working on the self'. It is this encouragement of self-improvement in the image of accepted norms of behaviour and action – the 'politics of the self' – that constitutes the 'active citizen' of neoliberal society, rendering them governable through the very forms of knowledge and practice that constitute our accepted norms. In this sense, a Foucauldian conceptualisation considers neoliberalism as government of the populace at the level of the individual body, as exercised through self-regulatory capacities of individuals and asymmetrical power relations spread throughout the social body and as immanent in the apparatuses of knowledge, discourse and practice that provide the very norms that guide our ways of thinking and acting. Thus, by targeting individual health through health surveillance and encouraging population well-being through individualised well-being practices, the post-1997 NHS reforms can be considered to legitimate the emergence of technologies in the image of this characterisation of neoliberalism.

The construction of 'well-being' that has been incorporated as a technology of neoliberal governance in the post-1997 policies positions the requirement for improvement on the individual, with forms of self-care considered to improve individual health and, thus, population health. However, the positioning of well-being as an outcome of engagement in forms of self-care is a relatively recently representation, one that has replaced well-being as collective measure of national stability and economic prosperity with an individualised, psychological and therapeutic understanding. As summarised by Sointu (2005), this can be seen to mark a shift from the 'body politic' – the well-being of the citizenry of nation states as constituted by national stability and economic prosperity – to the 'body personal' – well-being as relating to individual health, and as 'actively produced' by the individual through a variety of personal well-being enhancing practices. In this new 'actively produced' individual well-being, the citizen is still the focus, but the outcome is a form of government that encourages 'care of the self', allowing for state rollback of provision of health care for the citizenry.

Two policies that can be considered to have aided this shifting understanding of well-being as well as conditioning their emergence within the post-1997 apparatus of health are the Black Report and the Health Divide. Originally constructed and deployed as a means of problematising rising unemployment conditioned by the enactment of deindustrialisation, the recommendations legitimated by the report were enacted through the 'modernising agenda' of the New Labour government. The position constructed across the reports is that poor outcomes in health and well-being are related to structural and material inequalities across multiple domains, that these inequalities cause long-term trends in poor health mortality, and by intervening to reduce these structural and material inequalities, health and well-being outcomes of the populace would improve. However, the reports also construct the importance of increased health surveillance, promotion and prevention activities, and movement from individual institutional approaches to an integrated 'total' approach as key to solving the problem, as this would allow for the encouragement of 'good health among a larger proportion of the population' (Black, Morris, Smith, Townsend, & Davidson, 1988, p. 202).

The Function of Well-being and Neoliberalism in the Scottish Apparatus of Health

The discourses and technologies of well-being are prominent in Scottish government policies post-devolution from Westminster in 1999. Placed as a central aim of the newly devolved Scottish administration by the National Programme for

Improving Mental Health and Well-being, the achievement of mental health and mental well-being was positioned as the solution to Scotland's societal ills. The stated aim of this national programme of health improvement was to improve understandings of positive mental health to enable the Scottish public to take care of their *own* mental health, to help others, to *prevent* mental ill-health, and to promote awareness of where and how to access support and help when required. Children and young people were positioned as 'priority areas' for action (Black, Morris, Smith, Townsend, & Davidson, 1988, p. 2) by this national programme and, by not acting to promote their well-being, they were considered at risk of 'poor developmental outcomes' and increased 'mental health problems'.

Despite the lofty aim of population well-being improvement, the National Programme for Improving Mental Health and Well-being did not specify the approaches that would achieve its stated aims, only that they should met through collaboration between institutions such as the Education Department, schools, the NHS and 'others'. Through collaboration, well-being would be achieved by the 'development of effective front-line responses in schools for children and young people who experience emotional difficulties, mental health problems and mental illness' (Black, Morris, Smith, Townsend, & Davidson, 1988, p. 8). The lack of specificity can be considered to have allowed for a multitude of technologies to be invented through discourses of well-being, as was the case with the ADHD machine, allowing myriad problematisations to be targeted through deploying well-being promotion or enhancement as the aim. The breadth of domains that were to be governed through well-being is illuminated by the Scottish government 'indictors of well-being' (Safe, Healthy, Achieving, Nurtured, Active, Respected, Responsible, Included: SHANARRI) (See: Scottish Government, 2013) – allowing for the targeting of diverse 'risks', such as abuse; harm at home, school or in the community; poor learning; poor development of skills, confidence and self-esteem; neglectful family life and/or place to live; physical activity levels; and activities of responsibilisation, such as school or local community group involvement. These seven indicators are deployed in the construction of well-being across multiple policies and, more recently, have been codified in the Children and Young People (Scotland) Act (2014), allowing for well-being to be used to organise and make sense of every aspect of children and young people's lives and to govern these areas under the pretence of protecting their welfare.

As has been discussed by other authors (Brady, 2014; McLeod & Wright, 2016), and as has been illuminated here, there is not a coherent apparatus or single approach at work, but a particular governmental rationality that takes on different discourses and practices across time, space and problem; with government of young people, the discourse of well-being provides a space in which technologies of government can emerge. As is evident with the ADHD machine, the possibility of emergence is connected to multiple elements, conditioning its possibility, allowing it to be considered 'in the true' when it was first constructed as a 'proposal'. Through discourses of well-being, psychiatric knowledge was able to be reconstituted as well-being promoting: by intervening early, the

ADHD machine would promote well-being through reducing the impact of the risk of 'time' without a diagnosis and treatment, thus improving the life chances of children and young people. Additionally, the characterisation of ADHD as something that could be solved through school-based interventions alongside psychostimulant medication can be considered to reduce the 'seriousness' of a brain-based neurodevelopmental disorder to an educational disability that can be solved through school-based interventions, thus contributing to the promotion of well-being through increasing the potential for academic and educational attainment. The promotion or enhancement of well-being does not appear to be occurring, however – an irony here is the association of the diagnosis of ADHD with poor academic and educational outcomes; poor occupational, economic and social outcomes; and poor health-related outcomes.

These poor outcomes betray a silence within the current discourse of well-being and its deployment within the apparatuses that target young people – that well-being is a *requirement* of all young people and something that they must actively achieve. This requirement is made visible by the policies and guidelines regarding well-being: each one defines what well-being should look like and what the interconnected network of institutions must do if it is *not* being achieved. In this sense, well-being has become the expectation – all young people are expected to be well, to engage in activities that achieve this aim. Institutions act when there is at risk of it *not* being achieved: the strategic focus of apparatuses that target young people is to monitor all young people and step in whenever a risk exists to well-being, be that academic achievement, confidence, social skills, unemployment, lack of engagement with school and community. In effect, the range of areas of life that are targetable are infinite given the interconnection of the institutions that function as part of the apparatus, requiring only the vague notion of risk to well-being to enact procedures for its 'promotion'.

Extending the Machine: Creating an Everyday Practice of ADHD

The ADHD machine was run as a pilot project in one of the geographical localities that formed the wider region, before being 'rolled out' across the whole region in mid-2005; however, the approach was dissolved into the main referral system of the service in 2008, lasting three years as a speciality sub-service within the service. There was no indication of difficulties in the meeting minutes regarding the machine until an account of an 'extraordinary meeting' that was convened to discuss the 'problem of ADHD'; the problem in the account of the meeting was one of capacity, in that the ADHD machine was no longer able to manage the numbers of ADHD cases currently in the system or manage the number of referrals being received. The problem of capacity created by the machine related to the requirement for continued monitoring, by a professional with medical authority, for signs of the impact of the medication on physical growth, with all young people receiving medication required to attend 6–8 week 'medication reviews'. Procedurally, the reviews required measurement of height, weight and blood pressure of children and young people receiving medication in addition to the continued monitoring of the 'symptoms of ADHD'; as such, an outcome of the 'fast-tracked' approach of machine was an exponential rise in children and young people requiring monitoring of medication by the service.

Additionally, rather than reduce referrals, the ADHD machine conditioned the opposite through the creation of a system of relays for surveillance of young people by psychiatric knowledge and the expansion of psychiatric knowledge of ADHD into the school. The machine moved beyond its institutional boundaries, entering schools via a requirement for inter-agency collaborative working. This move into the school can be considered to connect educational professionals as relays in a system of psychiatric surveillance and judgement, thus increasing the purview of psychiatry and the availability of its knowledge within the school. However, the minutes of the extraordinary meeting do not attribute the increasing numbers of ADHD cases and referrals to an increase in psychiatric knowledge entering schools, or to the extension of the purview of psychiatry through the construction of relays of surveillance, or to the invention of a system for fast-tracked constructing of the ADHD child, but instead attributes this to a discovery of increased need. The explanation that appears to account for these effects is that the machine increased the skills and awareness of teachers and other educational professionals in recognising ADHD and that the need was much greater than was previously assumed. The logic deployed was that epidemiological studies indicate that ADHD is present in 5% of the under-18 population, whereas in this CAMHS region, prior to the ADHD machine emerging, prevalence of ADHD was only 0.4%, meaning that 4.6% of the region's under-18 population were 'undiagnosed ADHD'.

The solution to the problem created by the machine was to distribute the 'service ADHD caseload' across all professional groups that formed the multidisciplinary CAMHS team and to require each of these professional groups to perform a new streamlined approach as an individual clinical approach to ADHD assessment and diagnosis. In effect, the solution to the problem created by the ADHD machine was to 'mainstream' ADHD through the subjectivation, by psychiatric knowledge and practice, of multiple professional groups and approaches, thus creating an everyday practice of ADHD, an everyday psychiatric practice performed by all professional groups that would extend the process created by the ADHD machine.

Chapter 6

The Medication Review as Disciplinary Technology

As outlined in the last chapter, the initial step in this investigation was observation of ADHD clinical appointments. All the appointments I observed during my time in the service were 'medication reviews', which were presented as an integral part of the ADHD diagnostic process. Procedurally, the medication review consisted of a recurring six- to eight-week appointment and was framed as for monitoring the impact of treatment on 'symptoms' and potential side of effects of the treatment. Each of the sessions I observed followed the same format: a clinician from the 'ADHD team' conducted a clinical interview guided by an ADHD assessment 'proforma', where the presence of the symptoms of ADHD were located and quantified. Towards the end of the review, after completion of the clinical interview, the clinician took the young person to another room containing various medical 'tools' to measure their height, weight and blood pressure.

The rationale for positioning the first step in the investigation as the last chapter before concluding the document was because, after 'working backwards' from the starting point, I was unable to see the medication review according to how it was presented to me. Decontextualised from the wider apparatus conveyed across the previous chapters, the medication review can be considered as just that – a review of the impact of medication – but positioned within the wider apparatus, I was only able to see the medication review as a disciplinary technology, one that supported a wider strategic aim of producing a self-governing, self-improving young person.

The argument offered here draws on the work of Besley (2010) on the government of young people as 'risky subjects'. The argument put forward by Besley is that governmentality is, fundamentally, about the management of risk to the current and future functioning of the state through deployment of discourses and their technologies to manage social groups considered 'risky'. In this understanding, young people that cannot or will not control their conduct, cease to be 'docile bodies' and, thus, are positioned as problematic for state institutions. The outcome is that the state steps in to conduct their conduct through technologies of power, including interventions of the psy sciences, most often framed as about personal well-being, to promote forms of self-regulation and responsibilisation. These discourses and technologies are bound up with, and administered through, apparatuses such as, in the context of Besley's work, the youth justice system. In this investigation, it was not through a youth justice apparatus that the technology was deployed, but through apparatuses of health and education arranging around the strategic aim of promoting the well-being of every young person in Scotland. However, rather than being about the risk to the well-being of young people, the 'risk' being managed, as with Besley (2010), is considered to relate to the self-regulating capacity of the future adult citizen.

Framed from this perspective, the 'medication review' is considered a disciplinary technology within this wider apparatus. The observation that brought me to this conclusion was the requirement for monitoring the impact of medication on the 'symptoms' of the disorder. According to psychiatric knowledge, the - symptoms of ADHD are the result of faults in 'dopaminergic transmission' and 'serotonin transporter genes' (see: Manor et al., 2001). The 'treatment' – by psychostimulants such as Amphetamine, Dextroamphetamine and Methylphenidate – according to formal psychiatric knowledge, is considered to alleviate the symptoms by affecting the function and structure of the brain in relation to the specific abnormalities. The resulting 'therapeutic effect' is considered to be the reduction of inattention, impulsivity and hyperactivity, and resulting improvements in behaviour and social functioning (see: Greenhill et al., 2001). This improvement in symptoms did not appear to be a reality, however, emphasised by the continued visibility of 'symptoms' in each of the reviews I observed – these young people were receiving medication, had been for several years, yet were still displaying what were considered to be symptoms, which, for me, undermines the apparent effects and outcomes of treatment.

As such, the position taken in this chapter is that the ADHD machine, rather than assessing and diagnosing 'real' illness, produces ADHD by constructing a multiplicity of 'problems' through psychiatric power and knowledge, transforming them into ADHD, and allowing management through psychostimulant medication. The medication review can be considered part of this process. Through the ADHD machine, the young person receives a diagnosis of ADHD – a formal branding by psychiatric knowledge – and the medication review can be considered to hold this in place by continually subjectifying the young person through psychiatric knowledge. An additional function of the review is made visible when considered from this perspective – that the elements that structure it and its recurring frequency places the young person a modern-day space of surveillance and discipline in order to encourage self-regulation.

The Medical Examination as 'Ritual of 'Truth'

In the remainder of the chapter, I will elaborate the elements and functioning of the medication review according to Foucault's descriptions of disciplinary power. The aims of the chapter are to present the medication review as a 'ritual of truth' that produces the objects of knowledge used to fix ADHD on the young person, opening them up to constant surveillance and discipline through the medication review. My argument is that treatment by psychostimulant medication does not alleviate symptoms, but allows various 'problems' to be transformed into problems of inattention, impulsivity and hyperactivity, and managed, not through 'fixing' the faults in 'dopaminergic transmission' and 'serotonin transporter genes', but through a combination of medically induced docility and attempts at responsibilisation through psychiatric authority and knowledge. The role of medically induced docility was made clear in an interview with a psychiatrist. In the following excerpt, the discussion point was the connection of 'bad behaviour' with ADHD, despite this not being considered a 'symptom' of the disorder. The psychiatrist highlights that they would 'know' if the medication was working at a 'low dose', and how this 'low level' is often moved beyond as a means of medicating 'bad behaviour'. The origins of the 'problems' that are being medicated are then connected to the school:

> ***Psychiatrist:*** *That's the kind of what I do – the word pragmatic says it all. Whereas I think it's scary – you know – when you move environments because people kind of – but I wouldn't keep the children on medicine if it didn't work. I wouldn't ramp up to 150 and see if they blew up, or anything like that, you know? Because you can tell very quickly – very low levels – whether or not it's going to work. Because it's graduated. So at a low level it's going to work a wee bit, at the right level it's going to work better, you know?*
>
> ***Interviewer:*** *The thing that I've often been confused about with ADHD is – the bad behaviour thing. The reason for being here is often about bad behaviour. And the kind of increasing medication is because the bad behaviour is still around.*
>
> ***Psychiatrist:*** *I say to parents that this will – you know – that if this works it will improve your child's ability to attend, to bring the good behaviour to the table and the bad behaviour – and the bad behaviour is once we've improved their attention, their ability to learn new ways, and bring better skills to the table, is something that we need to look at using parenting approaches. A number of kids that I wouldn't dream of – it's a problem of the bad behaviour thing – it's bad behaviour, is it really not to do with your attention... Its executive function. And if you increase dopamine it makes them rigid and it actually contributes to their ability to argue. So you have to be very careful. It's actually – there's quite a low dose – there's always like a sweet spot. And if you go beyond it – and this is where I think zombie comes from –*
>
> ***Interviewer:*** *Right.*
>
> ***Psychiatrist:*** *– where people just keep going because they're trying to reduce their – medicate out the bad behaviour. And you're not going to medicate your way out of that.*

> ***Interviewer:*** *But this seems to be a thing that's become attached to ADHD – the main characteristic if you want, that's associated with young people considered to have ADHD.*
>
> ***Psychiatrist:*** *And if they don't have the behaviour, then they have really poor attention, they struggle to get the diagnosis. You know, you're right, a lot of people come here and people aren't coming and saying 'I think they're a wee bit inattentive' – they come and say – you know – 'behaviour is happening at school'.*

Before considering the elements of the medication review through this lens, I will offer an outline of the functioning of disciplinary power. This will then be connected to psychiatric knowledge and practice through Foucault's work on *Psychiatric Power* (2008), before being applied to what is considered to be a contemporary functioning of psychiatric power through the medication review.

Elaborating the Functioning of Disciplinary Power

Foucault's accounts of disciplinary power convey a configuration of power that functions through individualisation, surveillance and gathering information on the functioning of the human subject. The knowledge gathered is then deployable to induce certain forms of conduct and behaviour. The two main mechanisms by which it is enacted – hierarchical observation and normalisation – are considered to be fused in the 'examination'. Foucault outlines these mechanisms most clearly in *Discipline and Punish* (1979, pp. 170–194). Through hierarchical observation, individuals are made visible and knowable, allowing for their constant surveillance: the constant visibility is considered to function as a coercive force, allowing for transformation into docile and knowable subjects through an objectifying gaze (Foucault 1979, p. 172).

The coercive force of being made visible and knowable is considered to function through linkage with a normalising judgement. Being constantly visible allows for characteristics to be gathered and constructed into 'norms', ideals by which subjects can be continually judged against. The particulars of the expert 'gaze' form the particulars of the 'norm' – psychological gaze forms psychological norms, psychiatric gaze forms psychiatric norms, etc., – with each 'norm' providing a benchmark by which human subjects can be judged, and coerced towards, if outside of the parameters considered to form the normalcy constructed by the 'norm'. In this sense, 'norms' allow disciplinary power to 'correct': individuals can be compared to, and differentiated from, the wider population in accordance with set rules, which function to provide a 'minimal threshold' that they must achieve. This minimal threshold can be policed through application of means of surveillance and measurement, which act to constrain individuals, allowing for those falling outside the 'rules' to be positioned as outside the 'norm'. In short, normalising judgement allows disciplinary mechanisms to 'compare, differentiate, hierarchise, homogenise, and exclude' (Foucault 1979, pp. 182–183).

The final mechanism of disciplinary power, the examination, fuses observation and normalisation through looking and judging against constructed norms. Foucault describes the examination as a 'highly ritualised ceremony of power' (Foucault 1979, p. 184) which allows for the deployment of force, establishment of truth and the objectification and subjectification of the individual in accordance with the knowledge functioning as part of the mechanisms. The examination achieves this through visibility, documentation and the fixing of the individual as a 'case' (Foucault 1979, pp. 187–192). Through visibility, transgressions or movements from the norm are seen by the examining gaze, compared with the norm, classified as abnormal and the individual in need of intervention. The continual documentation of comparisons with the network of others that form the norm both contributes to the norm and fixes the individual as a case; they are objectified and subjectified by power functioning through knowledge, with each examination providing a snapshot, a moment in time, of the fabrication of the individual within a history of themselves, but a history determined for them by knowledge, power and the examining gaze.

In Discipline and Punish, Foucault contrasts the 'plague town' with the 'leper colony' as a means of highlighting the process of division, documentation and registration of population. For Foucault, the 'leper town' highlighted a process of exclusion through confinement, of exiling those marked as ill, making them unseen and forgotten, whereas, the 'plague town' highlighted a process of inclusion, surveillance and treatment by authorities. These two different, but not incompatible processes, are considered to have slowly come together, allowing for 'exclusion' within the wider population through analytical distribution and procedures of individualisation. This 'technique of power proper to disciplinary partitioning' was applied in spaces of internment, such as the 'psychiatric asylum' and the 'approved school', allowing control over individuals through division and branding, and coercive assignment and distribution (Foucault 1979, p. 199).

The panopticon is considered the exemplar of this configuration of power as it enabled, through its architectural components, both the exclusion and surveillance of inmates. Through a circular design, with cells facing inwards towards a central tower, inmates could be viewed at any point by both guards and inmates, with guards also in full view of the prison governor. The particular architectural arrangement of the prison allowed for constant surveillance without inmates knowing when they were under surveillance. The organisation of the components allowed for inmates to be differentiated into different classifications with application of means of training or correction enacted to encourage behavioural change towards a particular end. The 'major effect of this composition of disciplinary power is the inducement of a state of consciousness and visibility that assures the automatic functioning of power' (Foucault, 1979, p. 201) with the individual becoming the principle of their own subjection, accomplished through the internalisation of the gaze of authority being transformed into an internal gaze for policing and regulating the self.

The 'Actual' Functioning of Psychiatric Panopticism

According to Foucault, the perfect disciplinary institution functions as a 'microscope of conduct', 'an apparatus of observation, recording and training', which makes possible a 'single gaze to see everything constantly' (Foucault, 1979, p. 173). This is visible in the architectural feature of the 'ideal' of disciplinary power, the panopticon, with its circular design allowing for a constant gaze to make visible every aspect of the inmates functioning. But, as mentioned in Chapter 5, the actual everyday functioning of power does not adhere to an ideal, but in accordance with the limitations, blockages and resistances inherent within its actual application and functioning.

The panopticon was never built, but the elements that formed its disciplinary mechanisms were transposed onto various institutions, including the asylum. The outline of the functioning of disciplinary mechanisms within the asylum is offered in *Psychiatric Power* (2008). In this account, there is no 'central tower' for continual observation, but a system of relays of 'specialised' personnel that allowed for hierarchical continuous observation of disciplinary power. Foucault outlines the use of relays in the operation of the psychiatric disciplinary gaze within the asylum; the position of doctor is central to the operation of power within the asylum, but power operates because there are 'relays, networks, and reciprocal supports'; it is in this system of connections that power functions:

> [...] the figure himself [the psychiatrist] must function at first sight. But, in this first sight, which is the basis on which the psychiatric relationship is built, the doctor is essentially a body, and more exactly he is a quite particular physique, a characterization, a morphology, in which there are the full muscles, the broad chest, the color of the hair, and so on. And this physical presence, with these qualities, which functions as the clause of absolute dissymmetry in the regular order of the asylum, is what determines that the asylum is not, as the psycho-sociologists would say, a rule governed institution; in reality it is a field polarized in terms of an essential dissymmetry of power, which thus assumes its form, its figure, and its physical inscription in the doctor's body itself.
>
> But, of course, the doctor's power is not the only power exercised, for in the asylum, as everywhere else, power is never something that someone possesses, any more than it is something that emanates from someone. Power does not belong to anyone or even to a group; there is only power because there is dispersion, relays, networks, reciprocal supports, differences of potential, discrepancies, etcetera. It is in this system of differences, which have to be analyzed, that power can start to function.
>
> There is, then, a whole series of relays around the doctor, the main ones being the following. First of all, there are the supervisors, to whom Fodere reserves the task of informing on the

> patients, of being the unarmed, inexpert gaze, the kind of optical canal through which the learned gaze, that is to say the objective gaze of the psychiatrist himself, will be exercised. This relayed gaze, ensured by the supervisors, must also take in the servants, that is to say those who hold the last link in the chain of authority. The supervisor, therefore, is both the master of the last masters and the one whose discourse, gaze, observations and reports must make possible the constitution of medical knowledge. (Foucault, 2008, pp. 4–5)

The Functioning of Contemporary Psychiatric Power: The Review as Hierarchical Observation

Some to the 'elements' in the above account that allowed for psychiatric power to function through the asylum, arguably, are still at work in the modern functioning of the psychiatric disciplining gaze. This system of relays was very much visible in the medication reviews; from the 10 reviews that I observed, none were conducted by 'the doctor', instead being conducted by mental health nurses and mental health practitioners functioning as part of a network that included the doctor. The authority of the doctor was present in the conversations, however, being referred to by the clinicians conducting the reviews for various reasons. In the following excerpt of an interaction between a clinician, young person and parental authority figure, the clinician highlights the movement of knowledge of the young person between the clinician and the doctor, resulting in the 'intervention' being directed by the doctor:

> ***Clinician***: *So how's the symptoms been? How's things been in the morning? Do you know you need to take your medication in the morning when you get up – do you feel restless or anything?*
>
> ***Young person***: *No.*
>
> ***Clinician:*** *No? How about in the afternoons? How's the afternoons? Cos I see that Dr. M increased your medications in the afternoons. Has that been helpful?*
>
> ***Young person***: *I usually get tired in the afternoons.*
>
> ***Clinician***: *Right, OK. Take your medication OK?*
>
> ***Young person:*** *Yeah.*
>
> ***Grandmother***: *I think Dr. M increased it because you were getting very violent, weren't you? And mum was really worried.*

At the end of the session, when discussing the next appointment, the clinician again highlighted the role of the doctor, not only in disciplining the young person, but also in disciplining the 'practice' of the clinician conducting the medical review:

> ***Clinician:*** *Right. So, will I just take my lead then from Dr. M. Just looking – if you've seen him and then you feel that you need to come back to clinic, we can get you back in?*

Similarly, in the following excerpt, the authority of the doctor, this time the young person's GP, is invoked in a discussion regarding attendance at appointments for the medical review to take place, where the authority is deployed to urge engagement. The young person was to be transferred to an adult mental health service and the clinician was highlighting that the new 'adult services' clinician would not engage with the young person in the same way the child mental health service did (in a relaxed manner); in effect, if they did not attend their appointments, these would cease to be offered, resulting in the medication being stopped. The ending of medication is particularly pertinent to any welfare payments the young person is in receipt of in relation to the diagnosis.

> ***Clinician:*** *[...] you've GOT to make sure you attend appointments, and the appointments will probably be sent to you.*
>
> ***Young person:*** *Right.*
>
> ***Clinician:*** *Right?*
>
> ***Mum:*** *That doesn't mean bin them.*
>
> ***Clinician:*** *No. Because if you miss an appointment, they don't give you the kind of chances you get here. They will just say – you know – they've had a couple of offers of appointments, they haven't turned up, then that's like a discharge, and then you might have to wait longer next time. And then your family doctor might say 'oh, you've not been attending appointments, so you can't continue' [on medication].*

The Family as a 'Hinge' in the Functioning of Psychiatric Power

The excerpt above highlights another dimension to the functioning of contemporary psychiatric power: the family as a 'hinge' in the functioning of hierarchical observation. In the functioning of the asylum, the 'family' was an indispensable interlocking point, where the individual, rejected from various disciplinary systems, such as the school, as 'abnormal' and 'uneducable', was sent to be 'rehabilitated' in order to return to the school. The role of the family was to consign the individual to 'pathology' or 'delinquency', allowing for the asylum to take over and discipline through the knowledges and practices of psychiatry.

The medical reviews that I observed took place in the community, where the everyday practice of ADHD takes place. Young people are still admitted to the modern-day asylum – 'inpatient units' – but a diagnosis of ADHD (on its own) tends not to result in admission. This requires the modern psychiatric gaze to functioning without the physical authority of confinement within the walls of asylum. Arguably, the 'family' can still be seen to perform this 'interlocking point' in the functioning of contemporary psychiatric power, allowing for the management of young people without confinement and the walls of the asylum. The functioning of family in the asylum was described by Foucault as a 'cell within power' (Foucault, 2008, p. 79) functioning through the sovereign figurehead of the family (Foucault stated this as the father, but in the medical reviews, this was performed both by mother and father) monitoring the young person, relaying this information in the review, and enforcing the 'treatments' imposed.

This contemporary function of the family was visible in a number of the medication reviews, but also in interviews with education professionals. In the following excerpt, two teachers are discussing what supports would be put in place if a young person was having difficulties in the school. In the context of what supports would then be offered, one of the teachers highlights that parents often go straight to the GP for a diagnosis in order to determine the support that is offered:

> ***Teacher:*** *We'd try to find out about home circumstances, whether there's been any involvement from any other agency prior – you now – previous to coming here, or whether they are still ongoing. And initially it's an awful lot of extra information, because we're not equipped to make any judgments – we want to gather that bigger picture. And then we trial strategies and put things in place that we think might try and support that child. And it's only when – you know – you've exhausted strategies and they're not working do we then start to think we're going to need a wee bit of extra help, perhaps from [educational psychologist], to come and observe –*
>
> ***Teacher 2:*** *Often I think some of the parents have already gone to the GP and been to see some kind of support and perhaps already referred to CAMS. You know – so sometimes ... it comes in the other way.*

This was also recognised by an educational psychologist independent of the conversation with the teachers. In the following excerpt, the professional highlights the role of the family in bypassing the tiered-approach within schools and going straight to the GP seeking referral to CAMHS. The role of resourcing also figures in this excerpt; the professional highlights that what was once able to be offered as support within schools is no longer able to be offered due to cut-backs. In this context, families seek support in other ways:

> ***Educational psychologist:*** *I think just now we also seem to have a lot more parents going direct to their GP and asking for referrals directly. And again I think some of that is coming from there being just a lack of resource out there generally – you know – like the third tier, the voluntary sector – is pretty much gone. So there's a lot less supports out there that again previously might have taken us down different routes, that just aren't there. So parents are thinking 'where can I go', and they go to the GP and they get a referral straight in.*

The role of the family was not confined to fixing in place the forms of knowledge that would define and, thus, rehabilitate the problem; there was visibility in maintaining the diagnostic function once it was in place. In the following two excerpts, the family figurehead (mum) did not accompany the young person to the review, but the information was relayed to the clinician through a phone call prior to the review taking place. The young person in this interview was above 16 years old (hence attending unaccompanied by an adult), but the authority and functioning of the family figurehead and the information they add to the process is invoked with reference to the 'phone call' during the review:

Excerpt 1:

> ***Clinician:*** *So – when did I see you? A while ago?*
>
> ***Young person:*** *Quite a while ago.*
>
> ***Clinician:*** *March. OK. So there's been a bit happening. Your mum phoned up last month. When I saw you previously things were going OK. So firstly I just need to check – so we'll catch up on what, you know, your mum – about her phone call. What your concerns are. But just first off: still taking the medication?*

Excerpt 2 [later in the same review]:

> ***Clinician:*** *How are you finding it, focusing on the work and stuff like that at school?*
>
> ***Young person:*** *In the subjects that I enjoy it's easy, but... even, like, subjects that I don't enjoy, I feel the teachers know – they could ask like – I'm always there but I find it harder just sitting, ploughing through all the work.*

Clinician: *OK. So, sounds normal.*

Young person: *Yeah.*

Clinician: *Most of us would be like that. OK. And in terms of when your mum phoned, have things settled down since then? Because it sounded like things were quite heated then. Do you want to say a wee bit about what happened?*

Extending beyond the Confines of the 'Review'

To fully consider the functioning of power, we are urged to approach it as a 'multiplicity of force relations', with force considered as 'anything that influences the actions of individuals in a relation, that has an effect on their actions' (Foucault, 2007, p. xxii). This force can be 'immanent in a physical environment', in a 'social configuration', in a 'pattern of behaviour', in a 'bodily gesture', in a 'certain attitude' or in a 'way of life'. Thus, to fully consider the functioning of the medical review as disciplinary technology, the analysis needs to be extended beyond the review, to the wider elements of its apparatus, the various factors that work alongside the doctor, the network of relays and the family in the functioning of psychiatric power.

One such factor prominent in the review was the 'questionnaire': the medical review was a combination of 'clinical interview' and 'physical examination', with the interview being directed by an ADHD 'proforma'. Across all reviews, the same questions were asked, as each clinician followed the procedure laid out in the questionnaire. The questions related to the presence of 'symptoms' of ADHD, allowing for comparison against themselves, as a 'case', at different points in time. As outlined in the elaboration of disciplinary power, quantification of 'symptoms' also allows for comparison against a wider 'norm' and for judgement against normative parameters for 'correct' behaviours, forming the basis for corrective intervention. For this procedure to take place, however, there must be a 'norm' constructed from a wider network of individuals, from which comparison is made.

This was not the case with the medication review process. The questionnaire that guided the review was an internally constructed 'tool' and based on the characteristics of ADHD outlined by the *Diagnostic and Statistical Manual of Mental Disorders*, with quantification based on whether symptoms occurred 'never, sometimes, often, or very often'. My rationale for highlighting this is not to question the validity and reliability of the questionnaire; to do so would be to consider the questionnaire as an objective tool offering access to measurable traits, rather than as constructing the traits it claims to measure. Instead, the point being made is that I found the lack of reliance on normative information interesting as it highlighted the disciplinary function with the review as having moved beyond a requirement of normative information – ADHD was not quantified against a network of individuals, but solely against a quantification of the young person's behaviour across a history of medical reviews. The quantified 'symptomology' in this functioning can be considered to be a 'tool' within the disciplining process, with fluctuation used to urge self-governance, or as a basis for increasing dose to assist self-management through inducing docility:

> ***Clinician:*** *What about waiting your turn? Do you wait your turn for things?*
>
> ***Young person:*** *Sometimes.*
>
> ***Clinician:*** *Sometimes? What about forgetting day-to-day activities? Your day-to-day routine. Do you forget things that you're meant to be doing in your day-to-day routines?*
>
> ***Young person:*** *Not really. Apart from my medication.*
>
> ***Clinician:*** *So sometimes your medication!? Again, most people forget that. What about interrupting others when they're having a conversation – if your mum's on the phone or anything like that, you know? Somebody's talking.*
>
> ***Young person:*** *Only with my mum – all of us do that in our house, though.*
>
> ***Clinician:*** *Right. So sometimes with your mum. I'm just comparing it to the last time. So – I'm not sure if your mum was chipping in last time, or if it was mostly you. You seem a bit more – a bit more inattentive than the last time but not as hyper!*

Closing Down Alternative Discourse through Systematisation of Psychiatric Statements

The 'questionnaire' also appeared to serve another purpose – that of disciplining the clinician and governing what can be said about each young person. The same questions were asked by all clinicians across all medical reviews; questions inquired about sleeping and forgetfulness, but also in relation to concentration, fidgeting, keeping 'on-task', listening, running about/climbing on things excessively, etc. Each clinician moved through the questions in the same order, creating a uniformity of approach and response in each review; where deviation occurred, this was when examples were offered of behaviours that would indicate the presence of the symptoms being considered, but answers would always be quantified using the same scale outlined earlier. In the following excerpt, the procedure of two different clinicians is presented side by side to highlight the systematisation of procedure. The responses have been removed as it is the process and structure of the question that warrant consideration:

Clinician 1	Clinician 2
So there's fail to give close attention to details or making careless mistakes in schoolwork – you've not been at school much. But in that kind of thing, if you were having to concentrate or something, and you were having to pay close attention to, how's that been over the last week?	*Fail to give close attention to details or make careless mistakes in schoolwork? And feel free to chip in. What do you guys think about that? Is that never, sometimes, often?*
[…]	*[…]*
OK. What about fidgeting? You know, with your hands or with your feet?	*Very often? Right. What about fidgeting – hands, feet – or squirming in the seat?*
[…]	*[…]*
What about when you're – when you're doing something you're enjoying, or any task. Are you able to focus on that? Are you able to keep your attention on that – on that task? Or is it an issue?	*Very often. I'm observing about that. What about difficulties to staying attention on tasks or activities?*
[…]	*[…]*
Right. OK. If you were in class, or doing anything in the last week or two where you were meant to remain seated, would you be able to just sit on the seat – or would you be getting up when you're not meant to?	*In terms of in school and class – I don't know if you've heard – but is [young person] sitting down? Or is he up and down out of his seat when he's not meant to?*
[…]	*[…]*
OK. Do you listen to when you're spoken to directly? Do you always listen when you're spoken to directly like I'm doing just now?	*What about – does he not seem to answer when spoken to directly?*
[…]	*[…]*
Yeah? OK. Do you run about, climb on things excessively or when it's inappropriate?	*OK. So, certainly – it's often. But clearly, you're listening just now – So there is that – you know – that social communication about eye contact sometimes isn't there – but listening and picking it up. OK.*
	[…]
	What about running about, climbing things when it's not appropriate to do so? You know –

The questionnaires functioned to frame each young person's behaviour through ADHD knowledge, limiting different ways of talking about the behaviours and reducing the behaviour to a comparable number. Whilst each clinician and each young person talked about the object of each question in different ways (fidgeting, restlessness, etc.), the framing and quantification resulted in the same outcome, allowing for comparison of each young person with themselves over time, the fabrication of the ADHD subject through the categorisation according to the DSM symptomatology, and the continued use of psychostimulant medication and the medical review as disciplinary procedure.

Invoking Biomedical Authority: The Clinic Room and the Clinic 'Tools'

Another factor in the extended apparatus was the clinic room and the clinic 'tools': in each medical review, the young person was taken from the interview room to a medical examination room equipped with medical 'tools' for measuring weight, height and blood pressure. The room also contained a bed, wash basin, cleaning materials such as hand soap and paper towels, and was decorated in neutral colours. As mentioned earlier, the examination is considered a 'highly ritualised ceremony of power' (Foucault, 1979, p. 184); in the case of the medical review, an 'interview' is combined with a 'physical examination' in a highly ritualised ceremony: the examination took place at the same point in the medical review – at the end of the interview and before arranging the next appointment – and followed the same format – the young person was asked to follow the clinician to another room, was asked to sit on the bed and remove footwear, before height, weight and blood pressure were measured.

The measurement of these biological features was a procedure of each medical review, but in each of the reviews I observed, I did not hear an explanation offered as to why the measurements were taken. I later found out in general conversation that the measurements were taken to gauge whether physical growth was in line with predicted age-related norms, and whether blood pressure and pulse were elevated, in order to monitor for side effects of the medication. This was not how the physical examination was presented: the interactions between the clinician and young person were jovial and friendly, with conversation almost paternalistic (see excerpt below), which created a sense of interest in the well-being of the young person. The actual purpose for gathering the information, however, was to protect against the occurrence of known side effects of medication, thus protecting the functioning of the diagnostic process.

> ***Clinician**: OK. Well, I'll get your observations just and we can have a think about what next. So, bring the tape with us. We can see if you're still alive, yes?*
>
> ***Young person**: Ha, yes.*
>
> ***Clinician**: Pop your trainers off. If you can step on the scales – so, what have we got – 54 kilograms. Right, if you'd just put your head here.*

> ***Young person:*** *I don't think I've got anymore growing to do.*
>
> **Clinician:** *You might be. Still might be growing – so it's just about 170 centimetres, so that's just over five foot eight. This is indicating that you've taken quite a stretch.*
>
> **Young person:** *Finally! For about eight years now it's been the same.*
>
> **Clinician:** *You've grown an inch!*
>
> **Young person:** *Yes!*
>
> **Clinician:** *That's pretty incredible! And your weight's just up a wee bit – a kilo or so. Do you have sun tan lotion or something when you're outside? You're quite brown! 106 over 86 – that's fine. I'll just get your pulse. Super. Right, everything seems to be in order. So let's go back.*

Additionally, it could also be argued that an unintended effect of the physical examination is a rhetorical warranting of the procedure by biomedical discourse. ADHD is constructed as a neurodevelopmental condition by biomedical and psychological discourse; the condition exists in the neural circuitry of the young person's brain, with modernist scientific investigations giving this statement authority. Whereas, in the actual functioning of the medical review, there was no visible connection that bestow this authority; the presence of the condition is considered solely through the quantification of 'symptoms' by questionnaires. The addition of the physical examination, arguably, can be considered to function as a form of medical authority warranted through the use of 'tools' for measuring biological features, such as height, weight and blood pressure.

The medical authority bestowed on the review by the physical examination can also be considered to have been aided by the location and physical layout of the clinic in which the review took place. The clinic was located within a local community hospital, alongside medical services such as a minor injuries unit, an AAA (Abdominal Aortic Aneurysm) screening service, diabetes service, and an out-of-hours GP service. The child and adolescent mental health service (CAMHS) in which the medical review took place was originally housed in a Georgian townhouse that looked like, and was located amongst, local residential properties, but was relocated to the community hospital under the government procedures for identification and sale of NHS property (Scottish Government, 2011).

The new 'medicalised' location could be considered to further rhetorically warrant the review through invoking biomedical discourse: highly visible in the location were medical personnel in uniform, wheelchairs at the doorways, medical advice on walls, physically unwell patients with visiting relatives, clinical white décor, etc. The procedure for attending appointments added to this: young people had to walk through the location to a reception area for CAMHS visitors, the clinician was alerted to their arrival by a receptionist, who sat behind an enclosed space, conversing through a hatch only to take the particulars of the visitor. The young person was required to wait for the clinician in an open-plan, neutrally decorated, clinical waiting area. Once the clinician arrived in the waiting area, the young person was taken through a secured doorway into a corridor containing several doors indistinguishable from each other, then through one of these into the 'interview room'.

The procedure and space was similar to many other medical-related experience, despite being formed around a 'questionnaire' that could have been completed anywhere. Arguably, the familiarity of biomedical discourse invoked through the procedures just outlined bestowed a medical authority on the review – an authority imbued before the review even commenced through the space in which the medical review took place. In Foucault's account above of the functioning of the asylum, the figure of the doctor must function at first sight; 'the particular physique, characterisation, morphology, in which full muscles, broad chest, colour of hair, and so on' (Foucault, 2008, p. 4), impressing upon the patient the dissymmetry of the power relation. In the contemporary functioning of psychiatric power, the location of the 'medical review' can be argued to have taken the place of the functioning of the first sight of the doctor.

The (Paradoxical) Functioning of ADHD Knowledge and Treatment

The argument offered in this chapter is that the use of the ADHD diagnosis and psychostimulant medication is not about illness and alleviation of symptoms but the management of young people through normalising judgement and deployment of discipline as a means of encouraging self-responsibilisation. Several of the young people I met in medical reviews had been 'patients' in the Child and Adolescent Mental Health Service for over 10 years. The 'problem' that resulted in referral changed over the years they had been attending the service: for example, ADHD replaced 'the impact of domestic violence', 'depression', 'bed-wetting and single mother struggling to cope', 'speech and language difficulties', amongst other 'problems'. This also appeared to be continuing in the present moment: the 'problems' being discussed in the medical review included 'refusing to attend school', 'struggling to focus at work' [in a biscuit factory], 'difficulty adjusting to family reorganisation', 'not trying at school' [due to believing it was not worthwhile for future employment choice], and 'difficulty adjusting to the addition of a half-sibling to the family'.

Having being constructed as 'having' ADHD, all of these 'problems' were now being understood against the background of a 'biologically driven, brain-based neuro-developmental disorder', with all behaviours framed through the questionnaire considered to indicate the 'symptoms' of the 'disorder'. Through the process of construction, quantification and comparison, the young people in each of these reviews continued to be fixed according to this form of knowledge, allowing for ongoing construction of difficulties through the discourse of ADHD and, thus, legitimation as a target for 'treatment' with psychostimulant medication. But as mentioned earlier, the 'treatment' did not appear to alleviate the 'symptoms' – what was being constructed as 'symptoms' remained visible – its function appeared to be the legitimation of governance warranted upon medical authority exerted through a 'highly ritualised ceremony of power'.

Throughout the medical reviews, there were multiple examples of ADHD framing the 'problem' and its solution; the problem was placed at the centre of the review and questions were asked about fidgetiness, inattention, impulsivity, hyperactivity, behavioural difficulties, etc. and, through surrounding the 'problem' with these questions, the 'problem' was then reconstituted in these terms. Thus, common everyday issues, various irritations that occur daily, in being known through the medical review, came to be both produced by and reproducing of ADHD, thus excluding all other possible ways of knowing the difficulties. The questionnaire both functioned to govern the way the difficulties were known by limiting the way each clinician could question the difficulties and the way each young person could describe the difficulties, but also by constructing and quantifying the difficulties simultaneously as 'symptoms' of ADHD and, thus, as the 'result' of ADHD.

The parameters of normalcy governed in the medical review were difficult to pin down. There was no discernible norm or ideal against which governing took place, only the young person's own history as constructed by the clinical interview process. What was abundantly clear, however, was that the young person was to 'self-regulate' all forms of problematic behaviour. Arguably, the lack of any discernible limit of normalcy allowed for all forms of behaviour exhibited by the young person to be considered as ADHD and, thus, a problem of 'self-regulation'. This application of logic appeared to extend into all forms of living: in one of the medical reviews, the main focus was the young person's desire to be outside playing with friends and their lack of interest in returning home for lunch. The seriousness given to this as a problem of ADHD was confusing; it was not immediately clear why the parents were troubled by the young person's desire to be outside playing with friends. The main issue was not, however, about being outside, but the lack of interest in eating lunch. A side effect of psychostimulant medication is lack of weight gain or height growth (see: Ritalin Patient Information Leaflet, 2017, p. 8) and it was this concern that was framing the behaviour and the seriousness of this as problem of ADHD:

> ***Clinician:*** *So what had you experiencing some kind of anger or frustration?*
>
> ***Mum:*** *It's like – even just at eating times – meal times – when he HAS to do something that he doesn't want – I mean, whether it's just for eating or kind of going out, he's just 'Naah'.*

Young person: *And my appetite's not been that good. Like I'll feel hungry – then I ain't hungry.*

Clinician: *Right, OK. Because that was always something that was very good for you – your appetite.*
Young person: *Mhmm.*

Mum: *Aye. His appetite – I don't know whether it's he's not hungry or it's just that he's wanting to go out because it's nice. And the aggression's here because he's not getting to go out. He's having to stay in and eat and he doesn't want to do that.*

Clinician: *Right. So that's a change, because you always liked your meals.*

Young person: *Mhmm.*

Clinician: *You would eat all your meals and you usually had to eat your dinner, then you were going out. So how's that changed? Because you just don't want to eat anymore, or not as hungry?*

Young person*: It's just I don't feel that hungry any more.*

Clinician: *Right. Is that early on in the day? After you take your medication and do you start to feel hungry as the day goes on? So by tea time?*

Young person: *Yeah. I feel hungry but just then I'm not hungry.*

Clinician: *Right. Because sometimes you find that people struggle with their appetite during the day, but as the medication wears off, later on in the afternoon their appetite comes back, and you can eat normally.*

Young person: *At night I can maybe eat good.*

Clinician: *Right. So appetite at night – is that better than during the day?*

Young person: *A tiny bit.*

Mum: *No. If he can get to his friends, he refuses to eat. It's more like – I don't know whether it's the appetite or whether it's just that he's got more people he can play with now, and he just wants to do that.*

Clinician: *Right.*

Mum: *He wants to keep going all the time instead of taking time out to eat.*

Clinician: *Right. OK.*

Mum: *He'd rather take crisps and sweeties and run out the door or go to his pals and get a bag of chips when he's there. Because that way he can stay and he can do his own thing. I think the appetite's there – he's just not wanting to.*

The outcome here, and throughout the reviews, was that everyday common behaviours exhibited by young people, such as wanting to play with friends, come to be constituted as about ADHD, allowing for governance of the young person by the continued application of ADHD diagnosis and treatment. In the above interaction, being outside with friends and not returning for lunch was reconstituted from an everyday childhood occurrence to a 'risk factor' for weight loss and, thus, as a target for regulation. However, somewhat ironically, the regulation of this particular problem was to occur through self-regulation, with responsibilisation of the young person taking place through the deployment of strategies and techniques to shape the behaviour for a particular purpose (Rose, 1999); in this excerpt, it was to reduce the risk of weight loss through behavioural self-regulation:

Clinician: *Right. It might be helpful then to try and make a daytime routine during the holidays, like you would have for school.*

Young person: *Mhmm.*

Clinician: *That might be helpful. And then you know this is breakfast time, this is lunchtime, this is teatime – this is when I'm supposed to be in. Do you think that would be helpful?*

Young person: *Mhmm.*

Clinician: *And then you know – and then if your friends know they can come to the door at a certain time because then you'll have finished your lunch, or you'll have finished your dinner.*

Young person: *Mhmm.*

Clinician: *That would be better. And then there's not so much pressure on you and you're not going to be missing meals.*

Young person: *Yeah.*

Clinician: *Does that sound a bit reasonable?*

Young person: *Yeah.*

Mum: *As long as you keep to that when you go home.*

Clinician: *Well you would need to keep to that. I don't think that's unreasonable. I think that you as a young person, you have a good appetite, and we all know –*

Mum: *A great appetite.*

Clinician: *– he has. You've got a great appetite. You've got one of the best appetites of anybody I see here. You're my poster boy for eating your dinner. And I think it's a shame if that slips. And I get so much that you want to go out and be with your friends, and do all lots of different things, but if you say to them 'look, do you know what – I have to be in at – I don't know – what time's teatime at night? –*

Mum: *When [his brother] comes in from his working shift at half past eight.*

Clinician: *Right – so that's when you would have your evening meal, at half past eight?*

Mum: *Mhmm.*

Clinician: *Right. So that's not – you need to be able to say 'I have to be in because that's when I get my dinner'. When would you have lunch?*

Young person: *At lunch.*

Clinician: *Lunchtime? About one o'clock-ish? Yeah? So you say to your friends 'I need to be in from one o'clock to half past one to eat my lunch'.*

Young person: *Mhmm.*

Clinician: *'And I'll come out when I'm finished'. Then go out after your breakfast in the morning. That's not unreasonable. Yeah?*

Young person: *Mhmm.*

Clinician: *And then you're not getting frustrated, you're not feeling pressure from them to get out. But then you're not getting into arguments with mum either, because you're doing what you're supposed to be doing.*

Young person: *Mhmm.*

This responsibilisation of the young person – the shaping of a self-regulating subject through mechanisms of power functioning through ADHD discourse and knowledge – was not isolated to this medical review: it occurred for a variety of 'problems' across all medical reviews. For me, what is neatly highlighted in the above excerpt, is the main argument put forward in this chapter: that psychostimulant medication does not 'fix' the 'problem', instead allowing for continued surveillance and discipline of the young person through psychiatric knowledge and practice. The irony referred to earlier in the chapter, and inherent in the discontinuity with official knowledges and the everyday functioning of ADHD 'treatment', is that, according to the psychiatric explanation, the disorder signifies the presence of problems of self-regulation: the 'dysfunctional neural circuitry' that 'causes' the 'symptoms' of disorder implies that it is not possible to self-regulate. Yet here, and in every other one of medication reviews I observed, were young people, apparently suffering a disorder of self-regulation, being urged to solve the 'symptoms' through forms of self-regulation.

This paradox can be considered, rather than to highlight failure as 'medical treatment', to highlight the everyday practice of ADHD's success as a disciplinary technology. Receiving a diagnosis is the formal branding of the young person by psychiatric knowledge. The medication review can be considered to hold this in place by excluding other possible ways of conceptualising 'problems'. In this way, the medication review specifically, and the wider ADHD diagnostic process more generally, can be considered to function as disciplinary 'super-power' (Foucault, 1979, p. 271). Within the medication review, its procedures allow information to be gathered on the young person which then allows for their continued disciplining – the construction and quantification of 'inattentiveness', 'impulsivity' and 'hyperactivity' are used on a review-to-review basis as a means of legitimating continued application of the 'disorder' and 'treatment'. This reality, rather than being a failure, can be considered to indicate 'inverted efficiency' (Foucault, 1979, p. 271) where, rather than 'curing' ADHD, the procedures continually produce and reproduce ADHD young people, allowing for continued application of the knowledge and procedures as a means and mode of discipline.

The final element that provides the success of the procedure relates to what Foucault termed 'utopian duplication' (Foucault, 1979, p. 271). The everyday practice of ADHD, through its connection to public health/preventative discourses, allows for the continued practice of disciplining through the utopian ideal of promoting the well-being of *every* child and young person. However, the 'well-being' that is promoted is determined not by positive outcomes for the individual, defined by the individual, but by how well they fit with the wider aims and direction required of the populace. The everyday functioning of ADHD, and its continued practice, in this sense, functions as a governmental technology for achieving these aims. It continually 'fixes' 'risky' young people through notions of well-being and future social inclusion. The 'fixing' is presented as in their best interests: without the 'disorder' being fixed, they run the risk of being socially excluded through not having the skills and abilities for the future.

Chapter 7

Problematising ADHD through Micro-level Examination

This investigation sought to problematise the rising rates of ADHD diagnosis and resulting treatment with psychostimulant medication. Rather than engage with this problem by entering the 'battle over truth' that characterises much of the debate, this project adopted a critical sociological approach informed by Foucauldian and post-Foucauldian scholarship and contemporary transdisciplinary ethnographic research relating to subjectivity. This desire to avoid the battle over truth connects to my time as a practising clinical psychologist. I was often involved in 'battles over truth' at the level of the everyday, deploying arguments that highlighted the lack of validity and reliability of the 'evidence'; however, despite 'cancelling out' the evidence through critiquing its scientific rigour, the arguments did not appear to have any impact on the continued requirement for 'assessment of ADHD' within the child mental health services.

The battle I engaged in at the micro level of the everyday can be considered to be an enactment of the battle occurring at the level of official institutional knowledges. If one considers the knowledges that construct the 'literature' of ADHD, the battle is fought over the rules and procedures of 'objectivity' and 'methodological rigour', whereby studies that do not attend to these procedural requirements are deemed 'methodologically flawed. The outcome appears to be the 'cancelling out' of each position, most clearly articulated in the standoff between the 'International Consensus Statement on ADHD' (Barkley et al., 2002) and the 'Critique of the International Consensus Statement on ADHD' (Timimi et al., 2004). Despite this, diagnosis and treatment with stimulant medication continues apace: in Scotland, between 2002 and 2011, the increase in prescriptions was 105% (GROS, 2013) with Australia seeing an increase of 73% between 2000 and 2011 (Stephenson et al., 2012).

There is a silence betrayed in this battle over truth, both at the level of the everyday and at the level of institutional knowledges – one that, for me, makes the adoption of this approach as critique a pointless exercise. Despite highlighting that knowledge of ADHD does not conform to the rules and procedures that are considered to provide its scientific credentials, it continues to be dominant; so much so that it has become increasingly difficult to conceptualise young people, considered problematic within certain contexts, outside of this explanation. In short, the objects, concepts and procedural requirements of 'objective science' that legitimise ADHD as an object of psychiatric knowledge do not make any difference when deployed as a critique. The master's tools, it seems, do not dismantle the master's house (Lorde, 2018): the sheer force of the scientific truth value bestowed by the construction of ADHD by biomedical discourse appears to silence debate from within this discursive domain.

This point highlights the requirement for a different approach to the problem of ADHD – one that offers a critique, but from outside the frame of reference that provides its legitimacy. Such was my aim with this investigation. I wanted to understand how it was possible to *say* and *do* ADHD, for it to be *enacted*, in our present moment. My aim with this line of questioning was to simultaneously acknowledge its material existence and to reject the reality-version created by the knowledge and discourse that construct ADHD as a 'neurodevelopmental disorder'. For me, there was as much value in engaging in a critique that argues that it is 'not real' as there was in engaging in a battle over truth from within its frame of reference. It is very much 'real', but only in so much as it is enacted daily through the actions of multiple subjects located within an apparatus that is reinforced by, and reinforcing of, ADHD as a psychiatric disorder experienced by children and young people.

By considering ADHD in the way described above, I am following Rose (1999, p. x): it is commonplace for objects of scientific knowledges to described as 'not objective' and as 'socially constructed', especially in 'psy-sciences'. As he states, however, this is not particularly enlightening or useful – 'objects of thought are constructed in thought: what else could they be?'. So, as he suggests, a more useful approach would interest itself in questioning the ways in which objects are socially constructed; i.e., where they emerge; the authorities that are able to pronounce upon them; the concepts and explanatory regimes that construct them; the problems they solve, etc. The aim here is to understand how they came to be in place in the present moment – why these objects and knowledges, and not others, structure our reality – and to reveal the disreputable origins and unpalatable functions that have contributed to their emergence in the present moment.

This investigation is by no means the first to engage with ADHD in this way – e.g., Bailey (2013), Graham (2010) and Rafalovich (2004) – but where this investigation differs from what has gone before are the sites in which the investigation was conducted. Previous work, such as those above, has either adopted an archival approach, tracking the emergence of ADHD as an object of psychiatric knowledge or highlighted the construction and functioning of ADHD within schools or in education policy. These investigations are valuable, and much of what was carried out in this investigation was informed by them, but I wanted to take this investigation further by considering the connection between schools and mental health service in the construction of ADHD. As such, this investigation is unique – not only was it able to connect schools and mental health services, but it was able to provide an account of the functioning of procedures for managing young people considered problematic, at the level of their application, and to situate these within the changing discursive background from which they emerged.

In doing so, the investigation allows consideration of the application of 'actual' practice at the level of the young person. ADHD as an object appears 'monolithic' – or, certainly that it is how I experienced it in clinical practice and at the start of this investigation – possibly because of its rhetorical scientificness, continued exponential rise in application, and the 'global' reach of the knowledge that provides its visibility. These elements combine to provide ADHD with a 'realness' that is difficult to argue with, making it hard to know how to engage in critique: where does one begin with what feels like such an impenetrable reality? In this investigation, it was the micro level: the 'extremities of power' – the ultimate destinations, the regional and local forms and institutions, where it 'invests itself in institutions, becomes embodied in techniques, and equips itself with instruments' (Foucault, 1980, p. 96).

Approaching the investigation from the extremities of power allowed for penetration of the reality of official knowledges and access to the material effects they create in the everyday. What was revealed at this level was that the impenetrable reality of 'official' ADHD was nothing more than the production and reproduction of knowledge and discourse by various actors at various intersections of societal structure. At this level, the 'truth' of ADHD is not because 'objectivity' or 'accuracy of representation', but because of its usefulness in solving 'problems' within the apparatuses in which it is produced and reproduced in the present moment.

Combining Ethnography and Foucault to Investigate ADHD

The approach to this investigation aimed to reconnect the wider social, political and institutional factors that conditioned the possibility for the emergence of a particular form of ADHD-informed health care to be in place within an NHS region in Scotland in the present moment. An overarching aim was to consider ADHD from outside its dominant biomedical explanation as a means of critically questioning this explanation. By engaging with apparatuses (health and education) at a micro level, the aim was to reveal the interconnected nexus of elements in which ADHD functioned in the everyday, the 'problems' it solved and the effects conditioned by these solutions. From here, the aim was to 'work backwards', to provide a genealogical account of the pluralisation of events implicated in the eventual emergence of ADHD as the solution to the problems it solved. Procedurally, the aim was to question *how*, *why* and *where* 'young people' became a problem, how they were shaped as the problem they became, what possibilities were conditioned by constructing them as these types of problems, and to question how this changing background conditioned the current social practice of ADHD locally.

The approach described above was developed from Foucauldian and post-Foucauldian scholarship and contemporary transdisciplinary ethnographic research relating to subjectivity. In drawing on transdisciplinary ethnographic research, this investigation engages with subjectivity as both an empirical reality and an analytic category. By drawing on this form of scholarship, the understanding that informs this investigation is that subjects are 'epiphenomena': they are 'made up', constituted in and by technologies of knowledge and power

(Hacking, 1990, p. 3). From this position, subjectivity is considered to be multiple, mobile and externally constituted rather than a singular, fixed, internal 'natural essence' and, thus, requires analytical consideration of the external 'concrete constellations' in which it is continually shaped and reshaped.

Much of the ethnographic scholarship regarding subjectivity engages with the concrete constellations that shape subjectivity through examination of the ways in which people's inner states reflect the changing background of their everyday worlds. This particular focus marks a difference in this investigation, which was, for the most part, positioned outside of 'inner worlds' in the 'external concrete constellations'. As such, this investigation was influenced more by Biehl (2005), who, whilst working with the ethnographic consideration of the subject outlined above, focused more on the plasticity and malleability of reality; that is, 'the synthetic frameworks that mediate social control and recast concepts of a common humanity' (p. 16). In his investigation, the focus was 'subjectivity', but it was positioned as a 'material of politics' – the site upon which governance was enacted – with 'subjective reassemblage' continually occurring against a changing background of rational-technical politics and regional and local institutional responses (Biehl 2005, p. 16). The investigation, like this one, sought to make visible the apparatus of interconnections, and the broader social terrain from which they emerged, through which governance was enacted.

It was the particular understanding of the subject at the centre of the above application of the ethnographic approach that, for me, spoke to Foucauldian and post-Foucauldian scholarship – particularly those concerned with the study of governmentality. From a Foucauldian standpoint, governmentality refers to the complex of calculations, programmes, policies, strategies and tactics that shape the conduct of individuals: that which conducts conduct in order to achieve certain ends. However, government is more than just about controlling actions; it is also about constituting ways of thinking and acting, encouraging these through a wide range of political technologies and government-supported practices and institutions (e.g. laws, policies, interventions, initiatives, statistics and techniques), with the ultimate aim being the security and well-being of society.

In combining these approaches, this investigation positioned itself in the 'concrete constellations' that informed health and education practices and aimed to understand what made it possible for young people to be made into the ADHD subject; to be 'made up' as a young person 'with' ADHD and, thus, 'treatable' by psychiatric knowledge and medication. The investigation sought to understand this in the present – i.e., against what was ADHD being deployed as a solution? – but also historically – i.e., what made it possible for ADHD to emerge as a deployable solution? The aim here was not to provide a 'sociological description' of forms of governance, but an account of the pluralisation of events that made this way of governing thinkable and actionable in the present – the focus was on the ways in which 'young people' were divided, problematised and targeted across different periods and domains of life, the effects conditioned by these divisions and problematisations and how these effects are implicated in the production of the reality-versions that sustain their visibility. The investigation has attempted to make visible the conditions under which different ways of thinking about 'young people' were formed, the means of governance these ways of thinking legitimated, the effects these ways of thinking about and governing young people created, and the ways these effects have contributed to the shifting background upon which new ways of thinking and acting emerged.

Revealing Disreputable Origins and Unpalatable Functions

The starting point for investigation was observation of ADHD clinical appointments occurring in the present moment and then 'working backwards' from this point through various archival material, including clinical case notes, meeting minutes and current and historical policy. The 'inner worlds' of several health and educational professionals also formed part of the investigation, although this cantered on the procedural elements of their day-to-day practice rather than affect or beliefs. The narrative 'stepping-off' point of deindustrialisation and post-industrialisation was the end-point of working backwards from the present; but, as mentioned in Chapter 2, this is not where ADHD 'started' – it is where I chose to start the account, on the basis that 'social exclusion' had become a problem for schools to solve. The aim of starting at this point was to contextualise the 'things' that were problematised as 'social exclusion' – i.e., to make visible the conditions from which the 'things' (poverty, inequality, unemployment, health problems, social marginalisation, etc.) emerged and, thus, made them describable as 'social exclusion'. From here, I have attempted to provide an account of the multiple contingencies upon which the local practice of ADHD rests.

What was revealed was that, contrary to official institutional knowledges, the increasing visibility of ADHD was not conditioned by 'improvements in training', 'improved screening tools', 'better treatment regimens' or the 'accumulation of knowledge of aetiology' (see: Anastopoulos, Barkley, & Shelton, 1994; Lange, Reichl, Lange, Tucha, & Tucha, 2010; Mandell, Thompson, Weintraub, DeStefano, & Blank, 2005) but by a pluralisation of interconnected events conditioned by the enactment of deindustrialisation. Included amongst this pluralisation were wider 'elements', such as the shifting requirements of the young citizen and the emergence of technologies for achieving these requirements, the changing discourses of social exclusion and well-being, the widening parameters of the category of disability within educational discourse, and neoliberal reforms of health and education. More 'local' elements included the invention of technologies to 'support learning', widening health professional remits, and institutional responses to new requirements within the wider apparatuses of health and education. These are not offered as a singular ontological domain of practice, however, but as a multiplicity of elements, all with their own history, that have become connected in the production of the reality that allowed the ADHD machine to be acceptable as a solution at the point in time that it was proposed. In short, these elements can be considered to have created both the conditions for the ADHD machine to be thinkable and practicable and the intelligible background upon which its continued existence is legitimated.

An important feature of the investigation was locating what was considered to be unforeseen effects emerging from within interconnected elements and apparatuses. These unforeseen effects were what were considered to drive the continual displacement of apparatuses: I focused on these effects as 'problems' that were to be 'solved', with their construction as particular problems determining what was deployable as the solution. These effects can be considered to be multiple, interconnected and as shifting the strategic aims of the apparatus through the new requirements their construction as problems created. What was made visible in this investigation was a multitude of effects, including the production of inequality, poverty and unemployment, the requirement to continue in education, increased numbers of young people considered to require support to learn and increased referrals to child mental health services for assessment and treatment. The particular ways in which these effects were problematised determined what could be said about the problem that was constructed, what could be said and done about it and who was able to say and do those things. But the particular way in which 'effects' were able to be problematised was only possible because of the external relations of intelligibility offered by the wider elements of the apparatus described above. It is the interaction of effects created, the form their problematisation took, what this legitimated, how this was made a reality in the words and actions of individuals and the effects these words and actions created that are considered to drive the shifting background upon which thought and action takes place.

Using this theoretical frame, the investigation revealed increasing ADHD diagnosis as an effect of a 'solution' to local problems, within both the health and education apparatuses, with the solution made possible by the wider elements of the apparatus in which the problem emerged. Within health, increasing referrals, a requirement to promote 'well-being' and a requirement for integrated working with education (and other institutions) created the conditions in which the ADHD machine would function as a solution. Within education, social exclusion and the increased parameters of what could be constituted as a learning problem can be seen to have conditioned the possibility for the staged intervention approach and its 'space' in which 'support' from external agencies would function. This 'space', in which ADHD knowledge was able to function, can be seen to be conditioned not by the 'need' of the young person, but by the need of education to solve the problem of additional support needs within a context of increased 'demand' created by the requirement of 'inclusive' education to meet the needs of *every* pupil.

Rather than embodying 'equality for all', however, 'inclusive' education can be seen as a means and mode of governance of the young person. Education was revealed as a way of educating and shaping young people according to the requirements of a 'globalised' free market: they were positioned as the future adult and worker and, as such, required the necessary skills and abilities for the role. The school, supported by mental health and social services, was the means by which this governance was enacted, with the technologies of its enactment constructed as 'inclusive', as promoting 'well-being', and as reducing the likelihood of social exclusion and disadvantage through providing the skills to gain employment. Within these interconnected apparatuses, anything considered a 'risk' to future educational outcomes becomes a 'problem of learning' and, thus, targetable, first through education and then through mental health services. The problems of learning that I witnessed as part of this investigation that were constructed as ADHD were multiple, but *every single one of them* could be placed outside the young person within the structures in which they existed: poorly resourced schools, communities affected by poverty, lingering discourses that construct education as pointless, experience of abuse and trauma – these were all visible in the appointments I observed, but all were individualised as 'symptoms' of ADHD. The outcome, contrary to official knowledges and policy, was not reduced symptoms, improved educational outcomes and increased well-being, but the annulling of the voice of the young person through the continued fixing of their experiences as symptoms of ADHD by the medication review. The requirement: continued use of medication and the responsibilisation of the young person to improve *their* problem, rather than consideration of the context in which they came to be constructed as a problem.

How to Keep the Account Moving and Unfinished?

At the end of the introduction to *Vita*, Biehl (2005) highlights that an aim of the investigation was to bring forth the reality that was hidden behind *Vita* becoming the 'final line' for Catarina and to produce a form of knowledge that opened up a sense of anticipation in this most desolate environment (p. 24). He finishes with the question: how can the anthropological artefact keep the story moving and unfinished? This investigation shared similar aims: to bring forth the reality that was hidden behind the construction of young people as 'having' ADHD and to open up a sense of anticipation within the monolithic reality of ADHD. I also shared the desire to keep the investigation moving and unfinished. But how I might achieve this aim troubled me from the start of the investigation – how could I avoid bringing the investigation to a conclusion? What would be the purpose of not bringing the investigation to a conclusion? The requirement speaks to Mukherjee's precaution to avoid 'fatal unclutteredness' (1994, p. 6) when engaging in post-structural research. By doing so, one does not provide conclusions, but endings that recognise the temporariness and partiality of knowledge produced by post-structuralist investigations.

The temporariness of the knowledge produced through this investigation was starkly revealed very early in the project. As mentioned, I previously worked in one of the sites of this investigation. My recollection of the problem of ADHD from my time in the service was that it was a 'hot topic'; a debate that was engaged with vigorously by various clinicians in the service. One could say the battle over truth was fought daily. I fully expected the battle still to be raging, but it was not; in fact, ADHD did not seem to be a problem at all. What appeared to have taken over from ADHD was Autism Spectrum Disorder. This was visible in the clinical appointments I observed and in the conversations with the clinicians after appointments. The various behaviours of the young person being problematised in the clinical appointments were first constructed by ADHD, but subtler behaviours that did not 'fit' with the symptoms of ADHD were causally referred to as 'autistic traits'. This was also visible in the language of the educational psychologists, who would move between ADHD and ASD without qualification. Throughout the conversations with professionals from both sites, there was a sense of ADHD and autism being approached as the same 'problem', which was eventually confirmed in an interview with a consultant child psychiatrist. What appeared to have conditioned this shift was a 'treatment approach' within the service that was informed by the new category of Neurodevelopmental Disorders legitimated by the latest version of the *DSM* (V: 2013).

In this new category, the previous *DSM* (IV-TR: 2000) categories of Autism, Asperger's, Childhood Disintegrative Disorder and Pervasive Developmental Disorder Not Otherwise Specified were 'consolidated' into Autism Spectrum Disorder. ADHD was also added to this new category, whereas previously, it was situated within the category of Disruptive Behaviour Disorders. The combination of both disorder categories under the new term of Neurodevelopmental Disorders can be considered to position both as resulting from similar neurological dysfunction, which is what appeared to underpin the newly developed treatment approach within the service. In the approach, targeting parents and their parenting now functioned alongside administering 'small doses' of psychostimulants as the main treatment approach. The rationale offered for targeting parents of young people considered to have ADHD and ASD was that they needed to be 'super-duper parent[s]'. These parents needed to do the same things as other parents, but with greater resilience and consistency. The requirement of parents to be 'super-duper' parents was what appeared to legitimate the merging of both ASD and ADHD together under one approach:

> SMARTS is a parenting programme. And – you know – even with ASD and ADHD, I suppose, the parenting – you need to be a super-duper parent, in that you need to do similar types of things but with almost a greater level of awareness of when in timing, and a greater resilience, and a greater consistency. I just think splitting everything into bits has actually reduced our ability to help kids move forward, rather than increased and improved them. (Consultant child psychiatrist)

Within this new approach, medication would be used in small doses to improve attention as it would 'improve dopamine' in the 'attention' area of the brain. Small doses were considered to have the desired action and impact, while large doses, highlighted in the previous chapter by the same psychiatrist as causing the 'zombie effect', were considered not to work:

> *So in actual fact when you're putting kids on methylphenidate, you're putting them on the smallest amount of methylphenidate to improve dopamine in the attention area of the brain. You're just*

> *really – you're really dealing with the residual attention difficulty after you've resolved all the other issues. And I think we've got a bit confused about that. We tend to go straight in with methylphenidate and just ramp it up, and then wonder why it's not working.* (Consultant child psychiatrist)

The implication here is that psychostimulant usage would be reduced; however, this did not appear to be the effect created by the new approach. I was not aware of any young people's medication dosages being lowered. This was not present in the clinical appointments or the case notes. What was conveyed to me by teachers, however, was that there was an increasing visibility of young people being placed on small doses of psychostimulant medication without diagnosis, with medication being used as a 'tool' for assessment. The explanation that legitimated this appeared to connect the treatment approach outlined above: that the small dose would help reduce inattention and allow other 'symptoms' to be recognisable and treatable. In this new approach, the diagnosis of ADHD, whilst still fixed on the young people, was no longer required; medication was the starting point, which would assist in reducing neurodevelopmental disorder 'symptoms' and allow consideration of 'other' issues. In all of the conversations I had throughout the investigation, this new reality did not appear to be considered problematic, despite the awareness that the medication was not solving the 'problem':

Excerpt 1:

> ***Interviewer:*** *So that would be for the children who are already diagnosed?*
>
> ***Teacher:*** *Yeah, on ADHD diagnosis.*
>
> ***Teacher 2:*** *Or some other assessment – some children are being medicated but by no means are they kind of finished assessment, if you like.*
>
> ***Interviewer:*** *So they were medicated before diagnosis?*
>
> ***Teacher:*** *That's always happening now.*
>
> ***Interviewer:*** *Is that the case?*
>
> ***Teacher 2:*** *Absolutely.*

Excerpt 2:

> ***Teacher 1:*** *They've been given medication and for some days we actually need the medication to be in place to be able to*

> *assess the level of trauma that's around for some of these children. But we wouldn't have necessarily said ADHD in the way they're presenting within school. I think that's fair to say for a couple of children recently. We would have felt actually their trauma, their past and what they've been through, explains an awful lot of where they're at. But that seems to be coming back as a diagnosis and medication's been offered for these children. And it's varying degrees of success with it, I would say.*
>
> **Teacher 2:** *Yeah, well, there's one I'm thinking of at the moment who was diagnosed with ADHD with ongoing assessment with other – you know – queries – definitely other queries around possibly ASD – you know – and obviously that's ongoing. But [health professional] was saying, there's an idea of 'let's try and treat the ADHD part and let's see what happens'. That was what we were led to believe was the thing. So he's been, if you like, on medication since about June time, but actually what we see in class is still those hugely explosive outbursts – that anxiety, that – you know – and actually it doesn't – you're thinking 'has he had his medication? Is the medication working?'*

Does this delegitimise this investigation? I would argue that it does not and that the move from ADHD to ASD highlights the 'movement' that is central to the concept of the apparatus: that the changing background upon which thought and action takes place conditions what is possible, but also creates unforeseen effects that drive displacement and change in the apparatus. In this case, the new approach was conditioned by wider changes in formalised institutional psychiatric knowledge, but it was only acceptable locally because of the established reality of the ADHD constructed by the ADHD machine. Within the service, ADHD had come back under the purview of psychiatry due to the 'effects' created by the ADHD machine: the service 'case load' of ADHD was spread amongst all clinicians, but only for 'assessment'. Responsibility for diagnosis had returned to psychiatry, with medication reviews being conducted by nurses and mental health practitioners. The new system placed psychiatry central to the process, but with multiple connecting relays through which the new treatment approach would function.

This 'movement' also speaks to the second point above: the *partiality* of knowledge. By virtue of the displacement and movement, knowledge claims must be considered partial, never complete or fixed. In this sense, knowledge cannot be considered as being globally and trans-historically applicable; rather it is constituted by various actors at the various intersections of societal structures, and is continually dynamic. Through 'movement', but also through engaging with and producing knowledge, new frames are opened, give way, and in turn opens up new frames for engaging, theorising and acting (Olesen & Clarke, 1999). What is offered here, thus, is not considered trans-historically applicable, but as constructed through engaging with the apparatuses at the point in time at which I engaged. It is offered as a glimpse of a moving and changing reality, but also as means for engaging with the reality that has opened up through engagement and movement.

With the partiality of knowledge, we must also assume a second meaning: that knowledge can only ever be partial because of our embodied biases inherent in the 'way of seeing' that underpins our production of knowledge. The theoretical position adopted for the investigation positions the researcher (in this investigation, me) as within discourse and knowledge. We must consider ourselves as both objects and agents of knowledge, which requires us to consider the connections in which we are situated, what we see and do not see, what we produce and reproduce and how these things might function as part of the wider network of connections involved in the production of meaning. In this sense, much of what is produced by this investigation must be considered in light of my previous role in the service: how has this way of seeing influenced what I have produced here and what has remained silent? But I would also argue that this positioning is not necessarily a problem for knowledge production and that we should recognise, even celebrate, the role of our situated knowledges in the construction of knowledge. In this way, maybe what has been produced by this investigation could not have been produced if it were not for my previous position in the service. This certainly applies when considering the relatively unrestricted access that was available to me during this investigation.

So, What Are We To Do?

The points above can create an experience of 'paralysis'; or, certainly, that is something I experienced at points in the investigation: if what we produce can only ever be partial because of our inherent biases and the background upon which it was produced, forever being displaced, what grounds are left to stand on when making knowledge claims? I found Haraway's (1988) concept of situated knowledge particularly useful for moving beyond this paralysis. The problem posed by Haraway is whether we can have simultaneously 'an account of radical historical contingency for all knowledge claims and knowing subjects, a critical practice for recognising our own semiotic technologies for making meanings, and a no-nonsense commitment to faithful accounts of a 'real world', one that is partially shared and that is friendly to earth-wide projects of finite freedom' (p. 579). The premise informing the problem is that 'real' science is rhetorical, achieved through the enactment of illusionary objectivity-creating procedures, and that the knowledge claims are historically and culturally contingent. However, through this problem, and through a desire for a 'strong tool' for deconstructing the truth claims of science, critics have been left with no ground on which to stand when making knowledge claims of their own.

Within this context, Haraway offers an account of partial, 'situated' knowledges as forms of what she terms 'embodied objectivity' (p. 588). Using 'vision' metaphorically to describe embodied bias, she argues that *only* partial perspectives can offer an objective vision, which can only be produced through engaging with 'how we see'. What is urged here is engagement with partiality and situatedness: by engaging with both, we will 'see' what contributes to our unpacking of reality, but also allow for accountability of our knowledge claims through opening them up to critical examination. And by acknowledging our partiality and situatedness, we will avoid falling for the 'god trick': the idea that there is a disembodied, transcendent, conquering gaze from nowhere that allows access to an objective truth of our world. This form of seeing 'fixes' in place knowledge, closing down alternative reality-versions.

According to Haraway, faithful accounts of the 'real' world that are friendly to projects of freedom, modest meaning in suffering and limited happiness (p. 579) do not depend on a logic of discovery or an objective truth, but are 'partially shared' and depend on a critically informed, 'power-charged' conversation (p. 593). For me, acknowledging the partiality of the knowledge claims I have made throughout this book allows for the critically informed, 'power-charged' conversation to continue; and it is this continued conversation that will keep the investigation open and unfinished. The investigation is not finished, as the 'movement' above highlights; what is offered here is a partial account, one that urges for a continued examination of newly emerging reality of governance conditioned by the elements of the apparatus revealed by this investigation. Governance of young people (and other social groups) in accordance with certain aims continues; thus, critically informed investigations of its means and mode of functioning within the sites it meets its target must also continue.

Bibliography

Agamben, G. (2009). *What is an apparatus? And other essays*. Palo Alto, CA: Stanford University Press.

American Psychiatric Association. (1957). *Diagnostic and statistical manual of mental disorders*. Washington, DC: American Psychiatric Association.

American Psychiatric Association. (1968). *Diagnostic and statistical manual of mental disorders*. (2nd ed.). Washington, DC: American Psychiatric Association.

American Psychiatric Association. (1980). *Diagnostic and statistical manual of mental disorders*. (3rd ed). *(DSM-III)*. Washington, DC: American Psychiatric Association.

American Psychiatric Association. (2000). *Diagnostic and statistical manual of mental disorders*. (4th ed.). *Revised Text*. Washington, DC: American Psychiatric Association.

American Psychiatric Association. (2013a). *Diagnostic and statistical manual of mental health disorders: DSM-V* (5th ed.). Washington, DC: American Psychiatric Publishing.

American Psychiatric Association. (2013b). *Diagnostic and statistical manual of mental disorders: DSM-V*. Washington, DC: American Psychiatric Association.

Anastopoulos, A., Barkley, R., & Shelton, T. (1994). The history and diagnosis of attention deficit/hyperactivity disorder. *Therapeutic Care and Education*, *3*(2), 96–110.

Anderson, J. (1990). The 'new right', enterprise zones and urban development corporations. *International Journal of Urban and Regional Research*, *14*(3), 468–489.

Arcos-Burgos, M., Castellanos, F. X., Pineda, D., Lopera, F., Palacio, J. D., Palacio, J. D. et al. (2004). Attention-deficit/hyperactivity disorder in a population isolate: Linkage to loci at 4q13.2, 5q33.3, 11q22, and 17p11. *American Journal of Human Genetics*, *75*, 998–1014.

Armstrong, T. (1995). *The myth of the ADD child*. New York, NY: Plume.

Armstrong, T. (1996). ADD: Does it really exist? *Phi Delta Kappan*, *77*, 424–428.

Arnott, M. A. (2011). 'The more things change…?': The Thatcher years and educational reform in Scotland. *Journal of Educational Administration and History*, *43*(2), 181–202.

Atkinson, I., & Shute, R. (1999). Managing ADHD: Issues in developing multidisciplinary guidelines. *Australian Journal of Guidance and Counselling*, *9*, 119–127.

Bacchi, C. (2012). Why study problematizations? Making politics visible. *Open Journal of Political Science*, *2*(1), 1.

Bacchi, C., & Bonham, J. (2014). Reclaiming discursive practices as an analytic focus: Political implications. *Foucault Studies*, 17, 179–192.

Bacchi, C., & Goodwin, S. (2016). *Poststructural policy analysis: A guide to practice*. New York, NY: Macmillan.

Bailey, S. (2013). *Exploring ADHD: An ethnography of disorder in early childhood.* Abingdon: Routledge.

Bakker, S. C., van der Meulen, E. M., Buitelaar, J. K., Sandkuijl, L. A., Pauls, D. L., Monsuur, A. J. et al. (2003). A whole-genome scan in 164 Dutch sib pairs with attention-deficit/hyperactivity disorder: Suggestive evidence for linkage on chromosomes 7p and 15q. *American Journal of Human Genetics*, *72*, 1251–1260.

Bakker, S. C., Van der Meulen, E. M., Oteman, N., Schelleman, H., Pearson, P. L., Buitelaar, J. K. et al. (2005). DAT1, DRD4, and DRD5 polymorphisms are not associated with ADHD in Dutch families. *American Journal of Medical Genetics Part B (Neuropsychiatric Genetics)*, *132B*, 50–52.

Baldwin, S. (2000). Living in Britalin: Why are so many amphetamines prescribed to infants, children and teenagers in the UK? *Critical Public Health*, *10*(4), 453–462.

Barkley, R. A. (1990). *Attention deficit hyperactivity disorder: A handbook for diagnosis and treatment*. New York, NY: Guilford Press.

Barkley, R. A. (1991). *Attention deficit hyperactivity disorder: A clinical workbook*. New York, NY: Guilford Press.

Barkley, R. A. (1997). *ADHD and the nature of self-control*. London: Guilford Press.

Barkley, R. et al. (2002). International consensus statement on ADHD. *Clinical Child and Family Psychology Review*, *5*(2), 89–111.

Barry, N. (2005). New Right. In K. Hickson (Ed.), *The political thought of the conservative party since 1945* (pp. 28–50). Basingstoke: Palgrave Macmillan.

Baughman, F. A. (2012). Retrieved from http://www.adhdfraud.net/the-adhd-fraud-how-psychiatry-makes-patients-of-normal-children/. Accessed on August 2019.

Beckett, A. (2006). *Citizenship and vulnerability: Disability and issues of social and political engagement*. Basingstoke: Macmillan.

Bell, C., Howieson, C., King, K., & Raffe, D. (1989). The Scottish dimension of TVEI. In D. McCrone & A. Brown (Eds.), *The Scottish government yearbook, 1989*. Unit for the Study of Government in Scotland. Scotland: University of Edinburgh.

Bell, D. (1976). The coming of the post-industrial society. *The Educational Forum*, *40*(4), 574–579.

Besley, T. (2010). Governmentality of youth: Managing risky subjects. *Policy Futures in Education*, *8*(5), 528–547.

Biederman, J., Faraone, S. V., Monuteaux, M. C., Bober, M., & Cadogen, E. (2004). Gender effects on attention-deficit/hyperactivity disorder in adults, revisited. *Biological Psychiatry*, *55*(7), 692–700.

Biehl, J. (2005). *Vita: Life in a zone of social abandonment*. Berkeley, CA: University of California Press.

Biehl, J., Good, B., & Kleinman, A. (2007). *Subjectivity: Ethnographic investigations*. Berkley, CA: University of Californian Press.

Black, D., Morris, J. N., Smith, C., Townsend, P., & Davidson, N. (1988). *Inequalities in health: The black report and the health divide*. London: Penguin Books.

Blair, T. (1997). *Bringing Britain together*. Speech at Stockwell Park School, South London, 8th December. Retrieved from http://www.britishpoliticalspeech.org/speech-archive.htm?speech=320. Accessed on April 22, 2018.

Blanchflower, D., & Freeman, R. B. (1994). Did the Thatcher reforms change British labour market performance? *The UK Labour Market: Comparative Aspects and Institutional Developments*, *12*, 51.

Brady, M. (2011). Researching governmentalities through ethnography: The case of Australian welfare reforms and programs for single parents. *Critical Policy Studies*, *5*(3), 264–282.

Brady, M. (2014). Ethnographies of neoliberal governmentalities: From the neoliberal apparatus to neoliberalism and governmental assemblages. *Foucault Studies*, 18, 11–33.

Breggin, P. (1998). *Talking back to ritalin*. Monroe, ME: Common Courage Press.

Breggin, P. R. (2002). *The Ritalin fact book: What your doctor won't tell you*. Cambridge: Perseus Books.

Brocki, K. C., Forslund, T., Frick, M., & Bohlin, G. (2017). Do individual differences in early affective and cognitive self-regulation predict developmental change in ADHD symptoms from preschool to adolescence? *Journal of Attention Disorders*, 1087054717693372.

Brumariu, L. E. (2015). Parent–child attachment and emotion regulation. *New Directions for Child and Adolescent Development*, *148*, 31–45.

Buchan, J., & Evans, D. (2007). *Realising the Benefits? Assessing the Implementation of Agenda for Change*. The King's Fund. Retrieved from https://www.kingsfund.org.uk/sites/default/files/field/field_publication_file/realising-benefits-assessing-implementation-agenda-change-james-buchan-david-evans-kings-fund-30-july-2007_0.pdf

Burr, V. (1995). *An introduction to social constructionism*. London: Sage Publications.

Bussolini, J. (2010). What is a dispositive? *Foucault Studies*, 10, 85–107.

Bynner, J., & Parsons, S. (2002). Social exclusion and the transition from school to work: The case of young people not in education, employment, or training (NEET). *Journal of Vocational Behavior*, *60*, 289–309.

Carabine, J. (2001). Unmarried motherhood 1830–1990: A genealogical analysis. In M. Wetherall, S. Taylor, & S. J. Yates (Eds.), *Discourse as data: A guide for analysis* (pp. 267–311). London: Sage Publications with the Open University.

Care Quality Commission (CQC). (2013). *The safer management of controlled drugs: Annual report, 2012*. Care Quality Commission Publication.

Carnwell, R., & Daly, W. (2003). Advanced nursing practitioners in primary care settings: An exploration of the developing roles. *Journal of Clinical Nursing*, *12*(5), 630–642.

Cassidy, J. (1994). Emotion regulation: Influences of attachment relationships. *Monographs of the Society for Research in Child Development*, *59*(2–3), 228–249.

Castellanos, F. X., Lee, P. P., Sharp, W., Jeffries, N. O., Greenstein, D. K., Clasen, L. S. et al. (2002). Developmental trajectories of brain volume abnormalities in children and adolescents with attention-deficit/hyperactivity disorder. *Journal of the American Medical Association*, *288*, 1740–1748.

Cicchetti, D. (2016). *Developmental psychopathology: Maladaptation and psychopathology* (Vol. 3). Hoboken, NJ: John Wiley & Sons.

Cohen, S. (1979). The punitive city: Notes on the dispersal of social control. *Contemporary Crises*, *3*, 339–363.

Cole, M. (2008). Sociology contra government? The contest for the meaning of unemployment in UK policy debates. *Work, Employment and Society*, *22*(1), 27–43.

Collier, S. J. (2009). Topologies of power: Foucault's analysis of political government beyond 'governmentality'. *Theory, Culture & Society*, *26*(6), 78–108.

Collins, C., & McCartney, G. (2011). The impact of neoliberal "political attack" on health: The case of the "Scottish effect". *International Journal of Health Services*, *41*(3), 501–523.

Conners, C. K. (2001). *Conners' rating scales revised.* Multi-Health Systems, Incorporated. Retrieved from https://www.mhs.com/MHS-Assessment?prodname=conners3

Conrad, P., & Bergey, M. R. (2014). The impending globalization of ADHD: Notes on the expansion and growth of a medicalized disorder. *Social Science & Medicine*, *122*, 31–43.

Conrad, P., & Schneider, J. W. (1980). *Medicalization of deviance: From badness to sickness.* St. Louis, MO: Mosby.

Cousins, M., & Hussain, A. (1984). The question of ideology: Althusser, Pêcheux and Foucault. *The Sociological Review*, *32*(S1), 158–179.

Craig, D. (2003). Re-territorialising health: Inclusive partner- ships, joined up governance and common accountability platforms in thirdway New Zealand. *Policy & Politics*, *31*, 335–352.

Crisp, R., & Powell, R. (2017). Young people and UK labour market policy: A critique of 'employability' as a tool for understanding youth unemployment. *Urban Studies*, *54*(8), 1784–1807.

Dale, R. (1989). The Thatcherite project in education: The case of the city technology colleges. *Critical Social Policy*, *9*(27), 4–19.

Danermark, B., Ekström, M., Jakobsen, L., & Karlsson, J. C. (1997). Generalization, scientific inference and models for an explanatory social science. In B. Danermark, M. Ekström, L. Jakobsen, & J. C. Karlsson, (Eds.), Explaining society: Critical realism in the social sciences (pp. 73–114). London and New York: Routledge.

Danson, M. W., & Lloyd, M. G. (1992). *The enterprise zone experiment in Scotland: Strategic planning or crisis management?* Unit for the Study of Government in Scotland, University of Edinburgh.

Davis, E., Beer, J., Gligora, C., & Thorn, A. (2001). *Accounting for change in disability and severe restriction, 1981–1998.* Working papers in social and labour statistics (2001/1). Belconnen, ACT: Australian Bureau of Statistics.

de Mello, C. B., Rossi, A. S. U., Cardoso, T. D. S. G., Rivero, T. S., De Moura, L. M., Nogueira, R. G. *et al.* (2013). Neuroimaging and neuropsychological analyses in a sample of children with ADHD-Inattentive subtype. *Clinical Neuropsychiatry*, *10*(2), 45–54.

Deacon, B. J. (2013). The biomedical model of mental disorder: A critical analysis of its validity, utility, and effects on psychotherapy research. *Clinical Psychology Review*, *33*(7), 846–861.

Deacon, R. (2000). Theory as practice: Foucault's concept of problematization. *Telos*, *118*, 127–142.

Dean, M. (2015). Neoliberalism, governmentality, ethnography: A response to Michelle Brady. *Foucault Studies*, *20*, 356–366.

DeGrandpre, R. (1999). *Ritalin nation: Rapid-fire culture and the transformation of human consciousness*. New York, NY: W.W. Norton and Company.

Deleuze, G., & Guattari, F. (1987). *A thousand plateaus: Capitalism and schizophrenia*. Minneapolis, MN: University of Minnesota Press.

Deleuze, G., & Guattari, F. (2004). *A thousand plateaus: Capitalism and schizophrenia*. London: Continuum.

Demaine, J., & Entwhistle, H. (1996). *Beyond communitarianism: Citizenship, politics and education*. London: Macmillan.

Department of Education and Science. (1985). *Better Schools*. London: HMSO.

Department of Employment/Department of Education and Science. (1981). *A new training initiative: A programme for action*. London: HMSO.

Department of Employment/Department of Education and Science. (1986). *Working together – Education and training*. London: HMSO.

Department of Health. (1997). *The new NHS: Modern and dependable*. London: Department of Health.

Department of Health. (1999a). *Making a difference*. London: Department of Health.

Department of Health. (1999b). *Agenda for change: Modernising the NHS pay system*. London: Department of Health.

Department of Health. (2000). *The NHS plan: A plan for investment. A plan for reform*. London: Department of Health.

Department of Health and Social Security. (1980). *Inequalities in health: Report of a research working group*. London: HMSO.

Department of the Environment. (1980). *Enterprise zones: A consultation document*. London: HMSO.

Department of the Environment. (1982). *Monitoring enterprise zones: One year report*. London: HMSO.

Dreyfus, H., & Rabinow, P. (1982). *Michel Foucault: Beyond structuralism and hermeneutics*. Chicago, IL: University of Chicago.

DuPaul, G. J., McGoey, K. E., Eckert, T. L., & VanBrakle, J. (2001). Preschool children with attention-deficit/hyperactivity disorder: Impairments in behavioural, social and school functioning. *Journal of the American Academy of Child and Adolescent Psychiatry*, *40*, 508–515.

Dwyer, P. (2004). Creeping conditionality in the UK: From welfare rights to conditional entitlements? *The Canadian Journal of Sociology*, *29*(2), 265–287.

Early Intervention Foundation. (2015). *About EIF*. Retrieved from https://www.eif.org.uk/about. Accessed on December 2015.

Education (Scotland) Act. (1945). Education (Scotland) Act (1945). Retrieved from https://www.legislation.gov.uk/ukpga/Geo6/8-9/37/contents

Education (Scotland) Act. (1981). Retrieved from https://www.legislation.gov.uk/ukpga/1981/58

Education Act. (1981). Retrieved from http://www.legislation.gov.uk/ukpga/1981/60/enacted

Education Reform Act. (1988). Retrieved from http://www.legislation.gov.uk/ukpga/1988/40/contents

Edwards, J., & Trott, C. (1995). Education for citizenship in Key Stages 1 and 2. *The Curriculum Journal*, *6*(3), 395–408.

Faraone, S. V., Perlis, R. H., Doyle, A. E., Smoller, J. W., Goralnick, J. J., Holmgren, M. A., & Sklar, P. (2005). Molecular genetics of attention-deficit/hyperactivity disorder. *Biological Psychiatry*, *57*, 1313–1323.

Faugier, J., & Sargeant, M. (1997). Sampling hard to reach populations. *Journal of Advanced Nursing*, *26*, 790–797.

Finance Act. (1980). Retrieved from http://www.legislation.gov.uk/ukpga/1980/48/pdfs/ukpga_19800048_en.pdf. Accessed on July 08, 2017.

Findlay, R. (2005). *Modern Scotland: 1914–2000*. London: Profile Books Ltd.

Fingleton, E. (1999). In praise of hard industries. *The International Economy*, *13*(5), 52.

Fischman, A. J., & Madras, B. K. (2005). The neurobiology of attention-deficit/hyperactivity disorder. *Biological Psychiatry*, *57*, 1374–1376.

Fisher, S. E., Franks, C., McCracken, J. T., McGough, J. J. et al. (2002). A genome-wide scan for loci involved in attention-deficit/hyperactivity disorder. *American Journal of Human Genetics*, *70*, 1183–1196.

Foucault, M. (1972). *The archaeology of knowledge*. London: Tavistock.

Foucault, M. (1975a). *I, Pierre Riviere, having slaughtered my mother, my sister, and my brother: A case of parricide in the 19th century*. Lincoln and London: University of Nebraska Press.

Foucault, M. (1975b). Interview with Roger Pol Droit. In M. Morris & P. Patton (Eds.), *Michel Foucault: Power, truth, strategy* (pp. 109–147). Sydney: Ferral Publications.

Foucault, M. (1977). *Discipline and punish: The birth of the prison*. London: Allen Lane.

Foucault, M. (1979). *Discipline and punish. The birth of the prison*. New York, NY: Vintage Books, a division of Random House.

Foucault, M. (1980a). Power/Knowledge. In C. Gordon (Ed.), *Michel Foucault: Power/Knowledge. Selected interviews and other writings 1972–1977*. Brighton: Harvester Press.

Foucault, M. (1980b). *Power/Knowledge: Selected interviews and other writings 1972–1977*. London: Harvester Press.

Foucault, M. (1981). The order of discourse. In R. Young (Ed.), *Untying the text: A poststructuralist reader*. London: Routledge.

Foucault, M. (1982). Afterword: The subject and power. In H. L. Dreyfus & P. Rabinow (Eds.), *Michel Foucault: Beyond Structuralism and Hermeneutics*. London: Harvester Press.

Foucault, M. (1985). *Discourse and truth: The problematization of parrhesia. Six lectures given by Michel Foucault at Berkeley, Oct–Nov 1983*. Transcribed by J. Pearson. Evanston, IL: Northwestern University. Retrieved from https://www.cscd.osaka-u.ac.jp/user/rosaldo/On_Parrehesia_by_Foucault_1983.pdf

Foucault, M. (1986). *The use of pleasure. The history of sexuality*. R. Hurley (Trans.). (Vol. 2). London: Viking Press.

Foucault, M. (1988a). Technologies of the self. In L. H. Martin, H. Gutman, & P. H. Hutton (Eds.), *Technologies of the Self*. London: Tavistock.

Foucault, M. (1988b). The concern for truth. In L. D. Kritzman (Ed.) & A. Sheridan (Trans.), *Michel Foucault: Politics, philosophy, culture. Interviews and other writings, 1977–1984*. New York, NY: Routledge.

Foucault, M. (1991a). Politics and the study of discourse. In G. Burchell, C. Gordon, & P. Miller (Eds.), *The Foucault effect: Studies in governmentality*. Chicago, IL: University of Chicago Press.

Foucault, M. (1991b). Questions of Method. In G. Burchell, C. Gordon, & P. Miller (Eds.), *The Foucault effect: Studies in governmentality*. Chicago, IL: University of Chicago Press.

Foucault, M. (1994a). Michel Foucault. In M. Foucault & J. D. Faubion (Eds.), and R. Hurley (Trans.), *Michel Foucault: Power, The essential works, 1954–1984*. London: Penguin Books.

Foucault, M. (1994b). *Michel Foucault: Power. The essential works of Foucault: 1954–1984*. London: Penguin Books.

Foucault, M. (1996). What is Critique? In J. Schmidt (Ed.), *What is enlightenment? Eighteenth century answers and twentieth-century questions* (pp. 382–398). Berkeley, CA: University of California Press.

Foucault, M. (1997). Penal theories and institutions (Collège de France Lectures, 1971–1972). In A. Sheridan (Ed.), *Michael Foucault: A will to truth*. London: Routledge.

Foucault, M. (1998a). On the ways of writing history. In J. D. Faubion & P. Rabinow (Eds.), *Michel Foucault: Aesthetics, method, and epistemology. The Essential Works of Foucault 1954–1984* (Vol. 2, pp. 284–285). New York, NY: The New Press.

Foucault, M. (1998b). *The history of sexuality, Vol. 1: The will to knowledge*. London: Penguin.

Foucault, M. (2000). On the ways of writing history. In M. Foucault, J. D. Faubion (Ed.) & R. Hurley (Trans.), *Michel Foucault: Aesthetics. The essential works, 1954–1984* (pp. 279–297). London: Penguin Books.

Foucault, M. (2001). *Fearless speech*. Los Angeles, CA: Semiotext[e].

Foucault, M. (2003). Governmentality. In P. Rabinow & N. Rose (Eds.), *The essential Foucault: Selections from the essential works of Foucault, 1954–1984* (pp. 229–245). New York, NY: New Press.

Foucault, M. (2007). *Security, territory, population: Lectures at the Collège de France, 1977–1978*. New York, NY: Macmillan.

Foucault, M. (2008). *Psychiatric power: Lectures at the Collège de France, 1973–1974*. New York, NY: Macmillan.

Fox, N. A., Rubin, K. H., Calkins, S. D., Marshall, T. R., Coplan, R. J., Porges, S. W. et al. (1995). Frontal activation asymmetry and social competence at four years of age. *Child Development*, *66*, 1770–1784.

Fox, N. J. (1994). Anaesthetists, the discourse on patient fitness and the organisation of surgery. *Sociology of Health & Illness*, *16*(1), 1–18.

Fraser, N., & Sinfield, A. (1987). The Scottish labour force in recession. In D. McCrone (Ed.), *The Scottish Government Yearbook, 1987. Unit for the Study of Government in Scotland*. Scotland: University of Edinburgh. Retrieved from http://www.scottishgovernmentyearbooks.ed.ac.uk/record/22989

Furlong, A. (2006). Not a very NEET solution: Representing problematic labour market transitions among early school-leavers. *Work, Employment and Society*, *20*, 553–569.

Gamble, A. (1988). *The free economy and the strong state: The politics of Thatcherism*. Basingstoke: Macmillan.

Gaventa, J. (2003). *Power after Lukes: An overview of theories of power since Lukes and their application to development*. Brighton: Participation Group, Institute of Development Studies.

General Register Office for Scotland (GROS). (2013). *Population Estimates, Council and Health Board Areas: Estimated population by age and sex*. Retrieved from http://www.gro-scotland.gov.uk. Accessed on April 10, 2018.

Gergen, K. J. (1985). The social constructionist movement in modern psychology. *American Psychologist*, *40*(3), 266.

Gewirtz, S., Whitty, G., & Edwards, T. (1992). City technology colleges: Schooling for the Thatcher generation. *British Journal of Educational Studies*, *40*(3), 207–217.

Giddens, A. (1998). *The third way: The renewal of social democracy*. Cambridge: Polity Press.

Giddens, A. (2000). *The third way and its critics*. Cambridge: Polity Press.

Google. (2016). *Google Books Ngram Viewer*. Retrieved from https://books.google.com/ngrams/info. Accessed on May 01, 2016.

Gordon, C. (1991). Governmental rationality: An introduction. In C. Gordon, G. Burchell, & P. Miller (Eds.), *The Foucault effect: Studies in governmentality*. Chicago, IL: The University of Chicago Press.

Gottlieb, G. (2007). Probabilistic epigenesis. *Developmental Science*, *10*(1), 1–11.

Graham, L. J. (2008). From ABCs to ADHD: The role of schooling in the construction of behaviour disorder and production of disorderly objects. *International Journal of Inclusive Education*, *12*(1), 7–33.

Graham, L. J. (Ed.). (2010). *(De)constructing ADHD: Critical guidance for teachers and teacher educators. Disabilities studies in education* (Vol. 9). New York, NY: Peter Lang Publishing, Inc.

Greenhill, L. L., Pliszka, S., Dulcan, M. K., Bernet, W., Arnold, V., Beitchman, J. et al. (2001). Summary of the practice parameter for the use of stimulant medications in the treatment of children, adolescents, and adults. *Journal of American Academy of Child and Adolescent Psychiatry*, *40*, 1352–1355.

Hacking, I. (1990). *The taming of chance*. Cambridge: Cambridge University Press.

Hacking, I. (1999). *The social construction of what?* Cambridge, MA: Harvard University Press.

Hall, J. (1988). Interview with John Hall, main sponsor of Macmillan CTC in Middlesborough (BBC Radio 4, 19 October 1988). Cited in S. Gewirtz, G. Whitty & T. Edwards (1992). *City Technology Colleges: Schooling for the Thatcher generation. British Journal of Educational Studies*, *40*(3), 207–217.

Haraway, D. (1988). Situated knowledges: The science question in feminism and the privilege of partial perspective. *Feminist Studies*, *14*(3), 575–599.

Harold, G. T., Leve, L. D., Barrett, D., Elam, K., Neiderhiser, J. M., Natsuaki, M. N. et al. (2013). Biological and rearing mother influences on child ADHD symptoms: Revisiting the developmental interface between nature and nurture. *Journal of Child Psychology and Psychiatry*, *54*(10), 1038–1046.

Harpin, V. A. (2005). The effect of ADHD on the life of an individual, their family, and community from preschool to adult life. *Archives of Disease in Childhood*, *90*-(suppl 1), i2–i7.

Harris, J. (2002). Caring for citizenship. *The British Journal of Social Work*, *32*(3), 267–281.

Harvey, D. (2007). *A brief history of neoliberalism*. Oxford: Oxford University Press.

Hawi, Z., Matthews, N., Barry, E., Kirley, A., Wagner, J., Wallace, R. H. et al. (2013). A high density linkage disequilibrium mapping in 14 noradrenergic genes: Evidence of association between SLC6A2, ADRA1B and ADHD. *Psychopharmacology*, *225*(4), 895–902.

Healy, W. (1949). (Chair) Round table: Psychiatry and delinquency: Critical evaluations. *American Journal of Orthopsychiatry*, *19*, 317–341.

Hebebrand, J., Dempfle, A., Saar, K., Thiele, H., Herpertz-Dahlmann, B., Linder, M. et al. (2003). A genomewide scan for attention-deficit/hyperactivity disorder in an extended sample: Suggestive linkage on 17p11. *American Journal of Human Genetics*, *72*, 1268–1279.

Hebebrand, J., Dempfle, A., Saar, K., Thiele, H., Herpertz-Dahlmann, B., Linder, M. et al. (2006). A genome-wide scan for attention-deficit/hyperactivity disorder in 155 German sib-pairs. *Molecular Psychiatry*, *11*(2), 196–205.

Hellmer, K., & Nyström, P. (2017). Infant acetylcholine, dopamine, and melatonin dysregulation: Neonatal biomarkers and causal factors for ASD and ADHD phenotypes. *Medical Hypotheses*, *100*, 64–66.

Henriques, J., Holloway, W., Urwin, C., Venn, C., & Walkerdine, V. (1985). Changing the subject: Psychology, social regulation and subjectivity. *Sociological Review*, *33*(4), 807–809.

Her Majesty's Stationery Office. (1990). *Encouraging citizenship: Report of the Commission on Citizenship*. London: HMSO Publication.

Hill, M. (2003). *Understanding social policy* (7th ed.). Oxford: Blackwell Publishing.

Hills, J., & Stewart, K. (Eds.). (2005). *A more equal society?: New Labour, poverty, inequality and exclusion*. Bristol: Policy Press.

Honan, E. (2007). Writing a rhizome: An (im)plausible methodology. *International Journal of Qualitative Studies in Education*, *20*(5), 531–546.

Howe, G. (1978). *Liberating free enterprise: A new experiment*. Speech to the Bow Group, June 26. Margaret Thatcher Foundation. Retrieved from http://www.margaretthatcher.org/document/111842

Ideus, K. (1995). Cultural foundations of ADHD: A sociological analysis. In P. Cooper & K. Ideus (Eds.), *Attention deficit/hyperactivity disorder: Educational, medical and cultural issues*. Kent: The Association for Workers for Children with Emotional and Behavioural Difficulties.

Information Services Division (ISD). (2012). *Medicines for Mental Health: Financial years 2003/4-2012/13*. NHS Services Scotland Publication Report. Retrieved from www.isdscotland.scot.nhs.uk. Accessed onAugust 11, 2014.

International Narcotics Control Board (INCB). (2012). *Psychotropic substances: Statistics for 2011, Assessments of Annual Medical and Scientific Requirements for Substances in Schedules II, III and IV of the Convention on Psychotropic Substances of 1971*. United Nations, NY: United Nations Publication.

Jäger, S., & Maier, F. (2009). Theoretical and methodological aspects of Foucauldian critical discourse analysis and dispositive analysis. In R. Wodak & M. Meyer (Eds.), *Methods of critical discourse analysis* (2nd ed.). London: Sage Publications.

Johnson, B. (1981). Translator's introduction. In J. Derrida (Ed.), *Dissemination*. Chicago, IL: University of Chicago Press.

Jordan, B. (1989). *The common good: Citizenship, morality and self-interest*. Oxford: Basil Blackwell.

Jørgensen, M. W., & Phillips, L. (2002). *Discourse analysis as theory and method*. London: Sage Publications.

Joseph, J. (2000). Not in their genes: A critical view of the genetics of attention-deficit hyperactivity disorder. *Developmental Review*, *20*, 539–567.

Joseph, J. (2002). Adoption study of ADHD [Letter to the editor]. *Journal of the American Academy of Child and Adolescent Psychiatry*, *41*, 1389–1391.

Joseph, J. (2004). *The gene illusion: Genetic research in psychiatry and psychology under the microscope*. New York, NY: Algora.

Joseph, J. (2006). *The missing gene: Psychiatry, heredity, and the fruitless search for genes*. New York, NY: Algora.

Kalms, S. (1988). *Interview with Stanley Kalms, Chairman of Dixons retail chain and main sponsor of the Bradford CTC*. Radio 4, June 06, 1988.

Kaltiala-Heino, R. (2010). Involuntary commitment and detainment in adolescent psychiatric inpatient care. *Social Psychiatry and Psychiatric Epidemiology*, *45*(8), 785–793.

Kearns, A. (1992). Active citizenship and urban governance. *Transactions of the Institute of British Geographers*, *17*, 20–34.

Keller, E. F. (2007). Whole bodies, whole persons? Cultural studies, psychoanalysis and biology. In Biehl, J., Good, B., & Kleinman, A. (Eds.), *Subjectivity: Ethnographic investigations* (pp. 352–362). Berkeley, CA: University of California Press.

Kendall, G., & Wickham, G. (1999). *Using Foucault's methods*. London: Sage Publications.

Kleinman, A., & Fitz-Henry, E. (2007). The experiential basis of subjectivity: How individuals change in the context of societal transformation. In J. Biehl, B. Good, & A. Kleinman (Eds.), *Subjectivity: Ethnographic investigations*. Berkeley, CA: University of Californian Press.

Klerman, G. L. (1978). The evolution of a scientific nosology. In J. C. Shershow (Ed.), *Schizophrenia: Science and practice* (pp. 91–121). Cambridge, MA: Harvard University Press.

Knobel, M., Wolman, M. B., & Mason, E. (1959). Hyperkinesis and organicity in children. *Archives of General Psychiatry*, *1*, 310–321.

Kraepelin, E. (1913). *Psychiatrie: Ein lehrbuch* (8th ed.). Leipzig: Barth.

Kuntsi, J., Pinto, R., Price, T. S., van der Meere, J. J., Frazier-Wood, A. C., & Asherson, P. (2013). The separation of ADHD inattention and hyperactivity-impulsivity symptoms: Pathways from genetic effects to cognitive impairments and symptoms. *Journal of Abnormal Child Psychology*, *42*(1), 127–136.

Lange, K. W., Reichl, S., Lange, K. M., Tucha, L., & Tucha, O. (2010). The history of attention deficit hyperactivity disorder. *ADHD Attention Deficit and Hyperactivity Disorders*, *2*(4), 241–255.

Langley, K., Marshall, L., van den Bree, M., Thomas, H., Owen, M., O'Donovan, M. et al. (2004). Association of the dopamine D4 receptor gene 7-repeat allele with neuropsychological test performance of children with ADHD. *American Journal of Psychiatry*, *161*, 133–138.

Larner, W. (2000). Neo-liberalism, policy, ideology, governmentality. *Studies in Political Economy*, *63*(1), 5–25.

Levitas, R. (1996). The concept of social exclusion and the new Durkheimian hegemony. *Critical Social Policy*, *16*(46), 5–20.

Levitas, R. (1998). *The inclusive society? Social exclusion and new labour*. Basingstoke: Macmillan.

Levitas, R. (2005). *The inclusive society? Social exclusion and new labour*. Basingstoke: Macmillan.

Leys, C. (1985). Thatcherism and British manufacturing: A question of hegemony. *New Left Review*, *151*, 12.

Lipsky, M. (2010). *Street-level bureaucracy: Dilemmas of the individual in public service*. New York, NY: Russell Sage Foundation.

Local Government, Planning and Land Act. (1980). Retrieved from http://www.legislation.gov.uk/ukpga/1980/65/pdfs/ukpga_19800065_en.pdf. Accessed on July 08, 2017.

Loe, I. M., & Feldman, H. M. (2007). Academic and educational outcomes of children with ADHD. *Journal of Pediatric Psychology*, *32*(6), 643–654.

Lorde, A. (2018). *The master's tools will never dismantle the master's house*. London: Penguin Classics.

MacDonald, R. (1996). Welfare dependency, the enterprise culture and self-employed survival. *Work, Employment and Society*, *10*(3), 431–447.

MacNaughton, G. (2005). *Doing Foucault in early childhood studies: Applying post-structural ideas*. Abingdon: Routledge.

Madison, D. S. (2012). *Critical ethnography: Method, ethics and performance* (2nd ed.). Thousand Oaks, CA: Sage Publications Inc.

Mandell, D. S., Thompson, W. W., Weintraub, E. S., DeStefano, F., & Blank, M. B. (2005). Trends in diagnosis rates for autism and ADHD at hospital discharge in the context of other psychiatric diagnoses. *Psychiatric Services*, *56*(1), 56–62.

Mann, M. (1983). Nationalism and internationalism: A critique of economic and defence policies. In J. A. G. Griffith & A. B. Atkinson (Eds.), *Socialism in a cold climate* (pp. 184–206). London: Unwin Paperbacks.

Manor, I., Eisenberg, J., Tyano, S., Sever, Y., Cohen, H., Ebstein, R. P. et al. (2001). Family-based association study of the serotonin transporter promoter region polymorphism (5-HTTLPR) in attention deficit hyperactivity disorder. *American Journal of Medical Genetics, Part A*, *105*(1), 91–95.

Manpower Services Commission. (1981). *A new training initiative: A consultative document*. London: MSC.

Matthews, R. C. O., Feinstein, C. H., & Odling-Smee, J. C. (1982). *British economic growth, 1856–1973*. Oxford: Oxford University Press.

McLeod, J., & Wright, K. (2014). Inventing youth wellbeing. In K. Wright & J. McLeod (Eds.), *Rethinking youth wellbeing: Critical perspectives* (pp. 1–10). Singapore: Springer.

McLeod, J., & Wright, K. (2016). What does wellbeing do? An approach to defamiliarize keywords in youth studies. *Journal of Youth Studies*, *19*(6), 776–792.

Melrose, M. (2012). Young people, welfare reform and social insecurity. *Youth & Policy*, *108*, 1–19.

Meulen, E. M., Bakker, S. C., Pauls, D. L., Oteman, N., Kruitwagen, C. L., Pearson, P. L. et al. (2005). High sibling correlation on methylphenidate response but no association with DAT1-10R homozygosity in Dutch sibpairs with ADHD. *Journal of Child Psychology and Psychiatry*, *46*, 1074–1080.

Meyer, S. B., & Lunnay, B. (2013). The application of abductive and retroductive inference for the design and analysis of theory-driven sociological research. *Sociological Research Online*, *18*(1), 1–11.

Mill, J., Xu, X., Ronald, A., Curran, S., Price, T., Knight, J. et al. (2005). Quantitative trait locus analysis of candidate gene alleles associated with attention deficit hyperactivity disorder (ADHD) in five genes: DRD4, DAT1, DRD5, SNAP-25, and 5HT1B. *American Journal of Medical Genetics, (Series B, Neuropsychiatric Genetics)*, *133B*, 68–73.

Miller, P., & Rose, N. (2008). *Governing the present: Administering economic, social and personal life*. Cambridge, UK: Polity Press.

Millon, T. (1986). On the past and future of the DSM-III: Personal recollections and projections. In T. Millon & G. L. Klerman (Eds.), *Contemporary directions in psychopathology: Toward the DSM-IV* (pp. 29–70). New York, NY: Guilford Press.

Mitchell, N. (2004). *Attention deficit hyperactivity disorder (ADHD – the debate hots up in Western Australia [radio programme]*. In J. Carleton (writer) & N. Mitchell (producer) 'All in the Mind', 19th June, 2004 (Melbourne, ABC Radio National).

Mol, A. (2002). *The body multiple: Ontology in medical practice*. Durham, NC: Duke University Press.

Molina, B. S., & Pelham, W. E. Jr. (2014). Attention-deficit/hyperactivity disorder and risk of substance use disorder: Developmental considerations, potential pathways, and opportunities for research. *Annual Review of Clinical Psychology*, *10*(1), 607–639.

Montgomery, C. A., Wernerfelt, B., & Balakrishnan, S. (1989). Strategy content and the research process: A critique and commentary. *Strategic Management Journal*, *10*(2), 189–197.

Moon, G., & Brown, T. (2000). Governmentality and the spatialized discourse of policy: The consolidation of the post-1989 NHS reforms. *Transactions of the Institute of British Geographers*, *25*(1), 65–76.

Mort, F., & Peters, R. (2005). Foucault recalled: Interview with Michel Foucault (conducted in 1979). *New Formations*, *10*, 9–22.

Mukherjee, B. (1994). *The holder of the world*. London: Virago.

Nairn, T. (1970). Enoch Powell: The new right. *New Left Review*, *61*, 3.

National Curriculum Council. (1990). *Curriculum Guidance 8: Education for citizenship*. New York, NY: NCC.

National Institute of Clinical Excellent (NICE). (2008). *Attention Deficit Hyperactivity Disorder (ADHD): Diagnosis and management of ADHD in children, young people and adults*. National Institute for Health and Clinical Excellence, guideline: CG72.

Naysmith, S. (2013). Rigidity of Iron Lady's ideology aided the devastation of heavy industry in Scotland. *The Scottish Herald*, April 9. Retrieved from http://www.heraldscotland.com/news/13099505.Rigidity_of_Iron_Lady_s_ideology_aided_the_devastation_of_heavy_industry_in_Scotland. Accessed on August 25, 2018.

Nicholls, D. A. (2009). Putting Foucault to work: An approach to the practical application of Foucault's methodological imperatives. *Aporia*, *1*, 30–40.

O'Farrell, C. (2005). *Michel Foucault*. London: Sage Publications.

Office for National Statistics (ONS). (2011). *Labour Market Profile: NOMIS Official Labour Market Statistics*. Retrieved from https://www.nomisweb.co.uk. Accessed on October 06, 2013.

Olesen, V. L., & Clarke, A. E. (1999). Resisting closure, embracing uncertainties, creating agendas. In A. E. Clarke & V. L. Olesen (Eds.), *Revisioning women, health, and healing: Feminist, cultural, and technoscience perspectives* (pp. 355–358). New York, NY: Routledge.

Paterson, L. (1993). Local variation in the Scottish pilot projects of the technical and vocational education initiative. *Research Papers in Education*, *8*(1), 47–71.

Paterson, L. (1997). *Student achievement and educational change in Scotland*, 1980–95. Retrieved from http://ser.stir.ac.uk/pdf/14.pdf. Accessed on October 06, 2013.

Peltonen, M. (2004). From discourse to 'dispositif': Michel Foucault's two histories. *Historical Reflections/Réflexions Historiques*, *30*(2), 205–219.

Peters, M. A., & Besley, T. A. (2014). Social exclusion/inclusion: Foucault's analytics of exclusion, the political ecology of social inclusion and the legitimation of inclusive education. *Open Review of Educational Research*, *1*(1), 99–115.

Pickard, S. (2014). The trouble with young people these days: 'Deviant' youth, the popular press and politics in contemporary Britain. *Revue Française de Civilisation Britannique – French Journal of British Studies*, *19*(1), 91–122.

Pilgrim, D. (2007). The survival of psychiatric diagnosis. *Social Science & Medicine*, *65*, 536–547.

Powell, P., & Inglis-Powell, B. (1999). *Raising difficult children: Realistic behaviour management for difficult children including those with attention deficit / hyperactivity disorder* (3rd ed.). North Parramatta: Gouldian.

Pownall, H. (2013). Neoliberalism, austerity and the health and social care act 2012: The coalition government's programme for the NHS and its implications for the public-sector workforce. *Industrial Law Journal*, *42*(4), 422–433.

Prince, R., Kearns, R., & Craig, D. (2006). Governmentality, discourse and space in the New Zealand health care system, 1991–2003. *Health & Place*, *12*(3), 253–266.

Prior, P. (1997). ADHD/hyperkinetic disorder: How should educational psychologists and other practitioners respond to the emerging phenomenon of school children diagnosed as having ADHD? *Emotional and Behavioural Difficulties*, *2*(1), 15–27.

Rabinow, P., & Rose, N. (2003). *The essential Foucault: Selections from essential works of Foucault, 1954–1984*. New York, NY: The New Press.

Radcliffe, N., & Timimi, S. (2005). The rise and rise of ADHD. In C. Newnes & N. Radcliffe (Eds.), *Making and breaking of children's lives*. Ross-on-Wye: PCCS Books.

Rafalovich, A. (2004). *Framing ADHD children: A critical examination of the history, discourse, and everyday experience of attention deficit / hyperactivity disorder*. Lexington Books.

Raffnsøe, S., Gudmand-Høyer, M., & Thaning, M. S. (2014). Foucault's dispositive: The perspicacity of dispositive analytics in organizational research. *Organization*, *23*(2), 272–298.

Rankin, M., Fielding, N., & Reeve, G. (1990). *Active citizens: New voices and values*. London: Bedford Square Press.

Riddell, S., & Brown, S. (1994). Special educational needs provision in the United Kingdom: The policy context. In S. Brown & S. Riddell (Eds.), *Special*

Educational Needs Policy in the 1990s: Warnock in the Market Place (pp. 1–28). London: Routledge.

Ritalin Patient Information Leaflet. (2017). Retrieved from https://www.medicines.org.uk/emc/PIL.4093.latest.pdf. Accessed on April 01, 2017.

Rose, D., Vogler, C., Marshall, G., & Newby, H. (1984). Economic restructuring: The British experience. *The Annals of the American Academy of Political and Social Science*, *475*(1), 137–157.

Rose, N. (1984). *The formation of the psychology of the individual in England 1870–1939*. Unpublished PhD thesis, University of London.

Rose, N. (1992). Governing the enterprising self. In P. Heelas & P. Morris (Eds.), *The values of the enterprise culture: The moral debate* (pp. 141–164). London: Routledge.

Rose, N. (1996). *Inventing ourselves: Psychology, power and personhood*. New York, NY: Cambridge University Press.

Rose, N. (1999). *Governing the soul: The shaping of the private self* (2nd ed.). London: Routledge.

Rose, N. (2000). *Powers of freedom: Reframing political thought* (1st ed.). Cambridge: Cambridge University Press.

Royal College of Nursing. (2012). *RCN fact sheet: Nurse prescribing in the UK*. Policy and International Department, April.

Rutter, M., Tizard, J., Yule, W., Graham, P., & Whitmore, K. (1976). Isle of Wight studies, 1964–1974. *Psychological Medicine*, *6*(2), 313–332.

Scottish Education Department. (1977). *The structure of the curriculum in the third and fourth years of the Scottish secondary school (The Munn Report)*. Edinburgh: HMSO: Scottish Education Department.

Scottish Education Department. (1983). *16-18s in Scotland: An action plan*. Edinburgh: HMSO.

Scottish Education Department. (1986). *16+ in Scotland: The National Certificate*. Edinburgh: Scottish Education Department.

Scottish Education Department. (1988). *Setting new standards for all Scottish pupils*. Edinburgh: HMSO.

Scottish Executive. (2003). *National programme for improving mental health and well-being: Action plan 2003-2006*. Edinburgh: The Scottish Executive.

Scottish Government. (2003). *Moving forward! Additional support for learning*. Edinburgh: Scottish Government Publication. Retrieved from http://www.gov.scot/Resource/Doc/47021/0023972.pdf. Accessed on April 22, 2018.

Scottish Government. (2011). *NHS Scotland Property Transactions Handbook: CEL 8*. Retrieved from http://www.pcpd.scot.nhs.uk/index.htm. Accessed on April 07, 2017.

Scottish Government. (2013). *UNCRC: The foundation of getting it right for every child*. Edinburgh: The Scottish Government.

Scottish Government. (2017). *Statutory guidance: Standards in Scotland's schools etc. Act 2000*. Edinburgh: Scottish Government Publication. Retrieved from http://www.gov.scot/Resource/0051/00515736.pdf. Accessed on April 22, 2018.

Scottish Office Education and Industry Department (SOEID). (1999). *Social inclusion: Opening the door to a better Scotland*. Edinburgh: Scottish Government. Retrieved from https://web.archive.org/web/19990508193310/http://www.scotland.gov.uk/library/documents-w7/sima-00.htm. Accessed on April 22, 2018.

Scottish Parliament. (2004). *Education (Additional Support for Learning) (Scotland) Act*. Edinburgh: HMSO. Retrieved from http://www.legislation.gov.uk/asp/2004/4/pdfs/asp_20040004_en.pdf. Accessed on May 07, 2018.

Scottish Parliament Education Committee. (2003). *Passage of Education (Additional Support for Learning) (Scotland) Bill 2003*. SPPB 66. Retrieved from http://www.parliament.scot/S2_Bills/Education%20(Additional%20Support%20for%20Learning)%20(Scotland)%20Bill/BBV66_Vol1.pdf. Accessed on April 22, 2018.

Scottish Public Health Observatory (ScotPHO). (2008). *Health and Wellbeing Profiles*. Retrieved from http://www.scotpho.org.uk. Accessed on October 06, 2013.

Seidman, L. J., Valera, E. M., & Makris, N. (2005). Structural brain imaging of attention-deficit/hyperactivity disorder. *Biological Psychiatry*, *57*, 1263–1272.

SEU. (2004a). *The social exclusion unit*. SEU Publication, Office of the Deputy Prime Minister. Retrieved from http://webarchive.nationalarchives.gov.uk/+/http:/www.cabinetoffice.gov.uk/media/cabinetoffice/social_exclusion_task_force/assets/publications_1997_to_2006/seu_leaflet.pdf. Accessed on April 22, 2018.

SEU. (2004b). *Breaking the cycle: Taking stock of progress and priorities for the future*. SEU Publication. Office of the Deputy Prime Minister. Retrieved from http://webarchive.nationalarchives.gov.uk/+/http:/www.cabinetoffice.gov.uk/media/cabinetoffice/social_exclusion_task_force/assets/publications_1997_to_2006/breaking_report.pdf. Accessed on April 22, 2018.

Shanahan, A. (2004, May 30). Jumping on the victim bandwagon, *Sunday Telegraph*, p. 4.

Sheridan, A. (1980). *Michel Foucault: The will to truth*. London: Tavistock.

Sidhu, R. K. (2003). *Selling futures: Globalisation and international education*. Dissertation, The University of Queensland.

Silver, H. (1994). Social exclusion and social solidarity: Three paradigms. *International Labour Review*, *133*, 531.

Silver, H. (2010). Understanding social inclusion and its meaning for Australia. *Australian Journal of Social Issues*, *45*(2), 183–211.

Sinclair, J., Ironside, M., & Seifert, R. (1996). Classroom struggle? Market orientated education reforms and their impact on the teacher labour process. *Work, Employment & Society*, *10*(4), 641–661.

Slee, R. (1995). *Changing theories and practices of discipline*. Brighton: Falmer.

Smelter, R. W., Rasch, B. W., Fleming, J., Nazos, P., & Baranowski, S. (1996). Is attention deficit disorder becoming a desired diagnosis? *Phi Delta Kappan*, *77*, 429–432.

Smith, P. (1988). *The Scottish economy decline and response*. Unit for the Study of Government in Scotland, University of Edinburgh.

Social Exclusion Unit. (1999a). *Bridging the gap: New opportunities for 16–18 year olds not in education, employment or training*. Report by the SEU. Office of the Deputy Prime Minister. Retrieved from http://dera.ioe.ac.uk/15119/2/bridging-the-gap.pdf. Accessed on April 22, 2018.

Social Exclusion Unit. (1999b). *Bridging the gap: New opportunities for 16–18 year olds not in education, employment or training*. London: HMSO.

Sointu, E. (2005). The rise of an ideal: Tracing changing discourses of wellbeing. *Sociological Review*, *53*(2), 255–274.

Solanto, M. V. (1998). Neuropsychopharmacological mechanisms of stimulant drug action in attention-deficit hyperactivity disorder: A review and integration. *Behavioural Brain Research, 94*(1), 127–152.

Sowell, E. R., Thompson, P. M., Welcome, S. E., Henkenius, A. L., Toga, A. W., & Peterson, B. S. (2003). Cortical abnormalities in children and adolescents with attention-deficit hyperactivity disorder. *The Lancet, 362*, 1699–1707.

Sroufe, L. A. (2009). The concept of development in developmental psychopathology. *Child Development Perspectives, 3*(3), 178–183.

St Pierre, E. A. (1997). Methodology in the fold and the irruption of transgressive data. *Qualitative Studies in Education, 10*(2), 175–189.

Standards in Scotland's Schools etc. Act. (2000). Retrieved from https://www.legislation.gov.uk/asp/2000/6/contents

Stephenson, C. P., Karanges, E., & McGregor, I. S. (2012). Trends in the utilisation of psychotropic medications in Australia from 2000 to 2011. *Australia and New Zealand Journal of Psychiatry, 47*(1), 74–87.

Stewart, M. (1991). *Keynes and after* (3rd ed.). London: Penguin Books.

Still, G. (1902). The Goulstonian Lectures on some abnormal psychical conditions in children. *The Lancet*, 1 (12 April): 1008–1012; (19 April): 1079–1082; (26 April): 1163–1167.

Tait, G. (2001). Pathologising difference, governing personality. *Asia-Pacific Journal of Teacher Education, 29*(1), 93–102.

Tait, G. (2006). A brief philosophical examination of ADHD. In G. Lloyd, J. Stead, & D. Cohen (Eds.), *Critical New Perspectives on ADHD*. London: Routledge.

Tanner, J. M., & Buckler, J. M. (1997). Revision and update of Tanner-Whitehouse clinical longitudinal charts for height and weight. *European Journal of Pediatrics, 156*(3), 248.

Thatcher, M. (1980, May 21). *Speech to Conservative Women's Conference*. Retrieved from http://www.margaretthatcher.org/document/104368. Accessed on July 01, 2017.

Thomas, J. (1993). *Doing critical ethnography (Qualitative Research Methods Series 26)*. Newbury Park, CA: Sage Publications.

Timimi, S. et al. (2004). A critique of the international consensus statement on ADHD. *Clinical Child and Family Psychology Review, 7*(1), 59–63.

Timimi, S. (2005). *Naughty boys: Antisocial behaviour, ADHD and the role of culture*. Basingstoke: Palgrave MacMillan.

Visser, J., & Jehan, Z. (2009). ADHD: A scientific fact or a factual opinion? A critique of the veracity of attention deficit hyperactivity disorder. *Emotional and Behavioural Difficulties, 14*(2), 127–140.

Vogt, W. P. (1999). *Dictionary of statistics and methodology: A nontechnical guide for the social sciences*. London: Sage Publications.

Volkow, N. D., Wang, G. J., Fowler, J. S., Logan, J., Gerasimov, M., Maynard, L. et al. (2001). Therapeutic doses of oral methylphenidate significantly increase extracellular dopamine in the human brain. *Journal of Neuroscience, 21*(2), RC121–RC121.

Walker, K. (2004). *Pandora's box of ills*. Courier Mail, p. 14.

Walker, S. III (1998). *The hyperactivity hoax: How to stop drugging your child and find real medical help*. New York, NY: St. Martin's Books.

Walker, S. P., Wachs, T. D., Gardner, J. M., Lozoff, B., Wasserman, G. A., Pollitt, E. et al. (2007). Child development: Risk factors for adverse outcomes in developing countries. *The Lancet*, *369*(9556), 145–157.

Ward, M. (2016). Enterprise Zones. *House of Commons Library Briefing Paper*, 5942. Retrieved from http://researchbriefings.parliament.uk/ResearchBriefing/Summary/SN05942. Accessed on July 08, 2017.

Warnock, M. (1978). *Special educational needs: Report of the Committee of Inquiry on the education of handicapped children and young people*. London: HMSO.

Watson, C. (2010). Educational policy in Scotland: Inclusion and the control society. *Discourse: Studies in the Cultural Politics of Education*, *31*(1), 93–104.

Weir, A. D. (1988). *Education and vocation: 14–18*. Edinburgh: Scottish Academic Press.

Whitehead, M. (1987). *The health divide: Inequalities in health in the 1980's: A review commissioned by the Health Education Council*. London: Health Education Authority.

Willis, P. (1977). *Learning to labour*. Farnborough: Saxon House.

Wolcott, H. (1999). *Ethnography: A way of seeing*. Walnut Creek, CA: AltaMira.

Wolraich, M. L. (1999). Attention deficit hyperactivity disorder: The most studied and yet the most controversial diagnosis. *Mental Retardation and Developmental Disabilities Research Reviews*, *5*, 163–168.

World Health Organization. (1992). *The ICD-10 classification of mental and behavioural disorders: clinical descriptions and diagnostic guidelines*. Geneva: World Health Organization.

Index

Printed and bound by CPI Group (UK) Ltd, Croydon, CR0 4YY

13/09/2026

14961027-0007